THE COMPLETE GUIDE TO
NAVY SEAL
FITNESS

FEATURING
THE 12 WEEKS
TO BUD/S WORKOUT

STEWART SMITH, USN (SEAL)

Hatherleigh Press
An Affiliate of W.W. Norton & Co.
5-22 46th Avenue
Long Island City, NY 11215
1-800-528-2550
www.getfitnow.com

The use of the words Navy SEALs does not imply nor infer any endorsement, either explicit or implicit, by the United States Navy or the Navy SEALs.

Before beginning any strenuous exercise program, consult your physician. The author and publisher of this book and workout disclaim any liability, personal or professional, resulting from the misapplication of any of the training procedures described in this publication.

Hatherleigh Press titles are available for bulk purchase, special promotions, and premiums. For more information, please contact the manager of our Special Sales Department at 1-800-528-2550.

Library of Congress Cataloging-in-Publication Data

Cover design by Gary Szczecina
Interior Design by Fatema Tarzi
Photographed by Peter Field Peck with Canon® cameras
and lenses on Fuji® print and slide film

Printed in Canada on acid-free paper
10 9 8 7 6 5 4

THE COMPLETE GUIDE TO
NAVY SEAL
FITNESS

**LT. STEWART SMITH,
USN (SEAL)**

**PHOTOGRAPHY BY
PETER FIELD PECK**

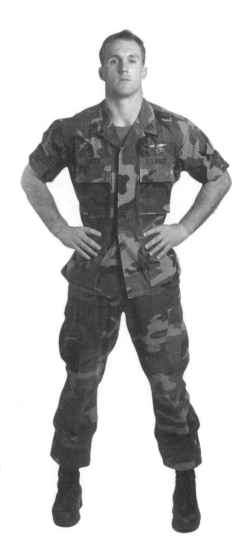

HATHERLEIGH PRESS

NEW YORK

Here's what readers are saying about
The Complete Guide to Navy SEAL Fitness:

"I used this book to help me increase my endurance, and boy did it ever do that. My push-ups are stronger, as well as my sit-ups, and my 2-mile went from 12:27 to a 11:50 in a matter of just 6 weeks."

—a reader from Honolulu, HI

"A great fitness book, not just for SEALs! Probably the best exercise routine yet. LT. Smith's book takes you from warm up to burn out in 12 weeks. The diagrams are clear and concise, and the program itself is time-efficient and, most importantly, successful. For those needing extra help or motivation, Smith himself presides over a posting board at the publisher's website."

—a reader from Guildford, England

"This is the best SEAL training book available. I've reviewed other SEAL training books and LT. Smith's is the best. The 4-week workout builds strength and stamina, leading to the 12-week workout.

"Very well documented and true-to-life book that delivers an honest and pure approach to SEAL training...Bottom-line: GET THIS BOOK IF YOU WANT TO FEEL STRONGER, MORE DISCIPLINED & READY FOR ANYTHING IN LIFE."

—a reader from Coronado Naval Base, CA

"Greatest SEAL training book I've ever read . . . If you want to make it through the training then this is the only book you will need. It tells you about BUD/S, who to contact, plus every exercise you will need to do."

—a reader from Massachusetts

"Great book! Worth its weight in gold. I started LT. Smith's workout three weeks ago and am feeling great. I liked the variety of exercise that it offers. You can feel the burn the first day. It's great . . . Just a good old-fashioned workout, except one hundred times more intense! Great book if you want to be a SEAL."

—a reader from Madison, OH

"One of the better all-around workouts available...Smith does more with less in this book. It is an excellent way to get into awesome shape. He covers all the basics in the book, and takes them to new levels. Definitely a book for those who are looking into the SEAL teams."

—a reader from Mountain Home, IDC

"Excellent book for those serious about getting in shape...This is an excellent book for those not wanting to deal with weights or machines. I suggest that you start with half the reps that the book suggests and build up. I've been using it for three weeks and I'm already seeing definition in my abs and upper body. Sometimes simplicity works best and this book is a proof of that."

—a reader from Birmingham, AL

"The best workout I have ever done. Not for the weak. This book has helped me improve my level of fitness to a higher level. I am currently in the third week of the twelve-week routine. I am training for the NYPD. I am sure that I will be successful, as I will be prepared both mentally and physically. This book was a life-saver."

—a reader from New York, NY

"An excellent book for the advanced athlete...this is an EXCELLENT book for those looking for a challenging workout. I highly recommend this book for those going into the military or those interested in law enforcement."

—a reader from Mankato, MN

DEDICATION

The Complete Guide to Navy SEAL Fitness is dedicated to those men who have chosen a profession most men would not dare...

To those men who do every day what most men would not dream of doing...

To those men who understand what it means to "never leave your swim buddy"...

And to those who have given their lives in the service of their country.

HOOYAH to the US Navy Frogmen past and present!

ACKNOWLEDGEMENTS

How do I begin to say thank you to the many people who have helped me in the past, who have shown me the right path to follow in life? I could fill several pages with names of family members, friends, SEALs, and other Naval Officers and Enlisted to whom I am grateful.

First and foremost—my family has been absolutely supportive in all the endeavors I have chosen. Thank you Mom, Dad, and Liz for always believing in me when the chances were slim that I would succeed. You gave me the strength to TRY, which has led to my SUCCESS. My wife Denise, who has been with me since I was a Midshipman, has given me the will and the desire to strive for excellence every day. Denise and my new child have given me the energy and motivation to prepare for the future by working hard today.

My best friend from my hometown of Live Oak, FL—Keith Bonds has and always will be a friend, no matter how long I am away. Through his steadfast friendship and comic relief, I have learned to enjoy life by relaxing and watching the Suwannee River slowly roll past. My best friend in the TEAMS, LT. Alden Mills, and I have been together since we met on restriction our sophomore year at USNA. Through BUD/S, Advanced Training, SDV Team TWO Task Unit Alpha, and who knows what else, he has always been there for me no matter what.

The enlisted men of the SEAL Teams have made a huge impact on my life. Their dedication to duty and their loyalty to their shipmates has made an unforgettable mark on my work ethic and enjoyment of missions accomplished. Thanks for your energy! I wish I could list all of you, but I risk forgetting one of the many of you who has been my swim buddy, point man, or a good friend. You know who you are. The many senior officers, who lead by example, have made an impression that will last a lifetime. To my mentor CDR Tom Joyce—I have learned so much from your leadership and your example of what a Navy family should be.

I thank God for giving me the ability to accomplish what I have. With the strength God has given me, I can only hope to help others achieve their personal goals. That is why I wrote this book—to receive the rewarding feeling of helping another reach their goals.

—STEWART SMITH

CONTENTS

PREFACE

The Complete Guide to Navy SEAL Fitness is a progressive, 12-week workout designed for individuals who are interested in becoming Navy SEALs or for people who like an extremely challenging workout. It is filled with pictures of stretches and exercises, running and swimming techniques, and a chapter on what to expect during SEAL training, as well as weekly workout charts that specifically guide you through some of the toughest workouts known. The unique concept of this workout regimen is that it requires no weight room equipment. You do not need to buy any equipment! All you need is a place to run, swim, and perform pull-ups and dips. Most school playgrounds or local parks have the necessary equipment.

This is the same workout that I perform with midshipmen at the US Naval Academy who attend Basic Underwater Demolition/SEAL Training (BUD/S) after graduation. Over thirty US Naval Academy graduates have used this workout and nearly all have had 100% completion records. This is a remarkable accomplishment, particularly when over 75% of BUD/S students traditionally quit.

Every year there are thousands of American teenagers who want to become Navy SEALs. There are also millions of Americans who want a challenging workout that does not require a membership fee. This workout not only physically challenges and prepares you for the toughest military training in the world, but also mentally prepares you by building your confidence and strength.

The Complete Guide to Navy SEAL Fitness also prepares you to ace the SEAL Physical Fitness Test (PFT) by measuring your fitness level every month as you take a practice SEAL PFT.

The Complete Guide to Navy SEAL Fitness starts at an intermediate level of fitness. In each of the first ten weeks, the exercise repetitions increase. The final two weeks taper off in order to prevent burnout from such high levels of intense training. I have also included a four-week "Pre-Training Phase" to help beginners build the strength and endurance that will be needed for the 12-week SEAL workout.

Chapters on how to run in the sand and swim with fins take this workout a step further. An elementary lesson on the sidestroke, the most common swim stroke at BUD/S, is vital if you are to successfully complete the 12-week training program. An instructional video on how to better your swim times for the SEAL PFT and how to swim with fins utilizing the uncommon sidestroke is also available.

If you follow and finish this 12-week workout, you will most likely find yourself in the best physical shape of your life. Finishing won't be easy, but with determination, you will make it. And wait until you see the results. Good luck!

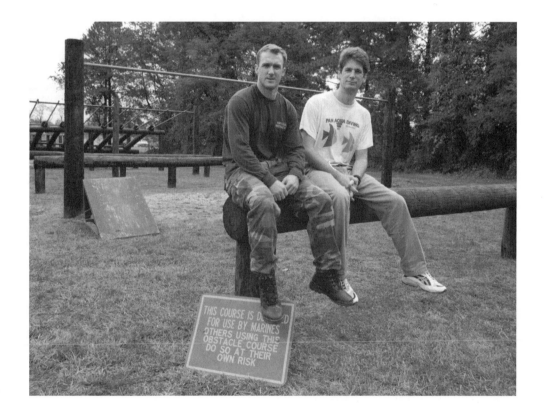

FOREWORD
TO THE REVISED EDITION

As with any product, time always wins out and things must be updated. I have added several new pages and a new chapter to the **Complete Guide to Navy SEAL Fitness.** Over the past three years, this book has helped hundreds achieve their dream of becoming Navy SEALs and helped even more become the fittest they have ever been. The workouts have been untouched in this revision, but the information about how to become a SEAL has been updated as well as the frequently asked questions page.

The Complete Guide to Navy SEAL Fitness is meant to be used two to three times in a year. That is only 24 - 36 weeks! In that time you will be amazed at the metamorphosis that occurs. After you have mastered this book, you may want to try **Maximum Fitness—The Complete Guide to Navy SEAL Cross-Training.**

FIVE PHASES OF FITNESS

If this is your first time picking up this book, here is the natural process of changing your life and becoming a new fit person.

1) Decision to get healthy / fit

Some will argue that it takes up to three to four weeks for something to become a habit. I say it takes three to four seconds! If you want to become fit, you will find every way possible to fit exercise into your schedule. Always remember, something is better than nothing. There will be days when you just do not have time to exercise an entire hour. Ten to fifteen minutes is better than doing nothing at all, so do some jumping jacks, pushups and stretches.

2) Doubt yourself

It is absolutely natural to have doubts about what you are undertaking. My advice is to start doubting yourself as quickly as possible and get over it. Realize that self doubt is a natural part of the process of becoming fit and face it and move on. Even SEAL trainees doubt themselves, but those who conquer doubt become members of the elite Navy SEALs.

3) Conquer doubt

Now you have conquered doubt—you can do anything you set your mind to —is what you just told yourself. This is where the mind and body connect. Use the physical workouts to be a catalyst to energize other areas of your life: work, relationships, school. I am a firm believer that exercising your body gives you the stamina and endurance to exercise your mind, spirit and relationships to others around you.

4) Associate yourself with fit and healthy people

Now you are fit, you are comfortable in settings with young and fit people. Your example will inspire others to want to be like you. Your confidence in yourself will increase and open doors for you that you never imagined. People will be amazed by your work ethic at work and at play. Eating healthy is now a habit for you. In fact, eating fast food makes you feel slightly "ill".

5) Conquer a goal for yourself—whatever you like to do—run, swim, bike, weight lift or calisthenics—set a goal to do any of the below or your choice...Try them all too.

RUN	SWIM	BIKE	WEIGHTS	PULL/PUSH/SITUPS
1) 5K	500 yd test	20 miles	100lb bench	5/50/50
2) 10 K	1000 yd test	50 miles	200lb bench	10/60/60
3) 10 mile	1 mile swim	100 miles	300 lb bench	15/75 /75
4) ½marathon	2 mile swim	Cross state	400 lb bench	20/100/100
5) marathon	3 mile swim	Cross Country	400+ bench	25+/120+/120+

5+) Mix all three: triathlon/iron man

Choose one or more categories of events and see if you can become a Fitness Grand Master with the author. Stew Smith's PT club at www.stewsmith.com and www.getfitnow.com

INJURY DISCLAIMER

Before beginning any strenuous exercise program, consult your physician. The author and publisher of **The Complete Guide to Navy SEAL Fitness** disclaim any liability, personal or professional, resulting from the misapplication of any of the training procedures described in this publication. Take your health and fitness seriously!

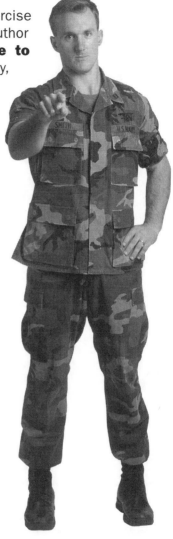

INTRODUCTION

THIS WORKOUT *WILL* PREPARE YOU FOR
SEAL TRAINING *OR* ANYTHING ELSE!

Any well-conditioned person can do these workouts. There are over 70 different combinations of workouts included in this book, with pictures of stretches, exercises, running, and swimming. Over 150 pictures teach you every exercise as well as the proper techniques for running, swimming, and training with the world's fittest individuals—The US Navy SEALs!

You might ask, how does this workout prepare me for anything else? Believe it or not, if you can successfully complete this 12-week workout challenge, you will be physically prepared for ANY other military training. From Basic training—Army, Navy, Air Force, Marine Corps—to advanced military training like BUD/S, this workout will physically prepare you to do them all! Even if you have no desire to be in the military, but enjoy working out every day, **The Complete Guide to Navy SEAL Fitness** will definitely get you into top physical condition.

More importantly, the unbelievable amount of confidence you will gain in your abilities will change your life. Never before have you been able to do 750 pushups in one workout or complete the exhausting four-mile-run-one-mile-swim-three-mile-run in an hour and a half, but with this progressive step-by-step exercise program you will be conquering what you thought was impossible. You have no idea how this will affect your personal and professional life! You will gain confidence in your abilities that people will notice. Your boss, friends, and co-workers will see a lean, fit, self-assured person who has the attitude that anything can be accomplished. You will feel like you have never felt before in your life. You will have the energy to work all day, come home, play with the kids, or do whatever else needs to be done.

Let's face it. First impressions are lasting impressions. When you walk into a room full of people, the first thing they notice is your appearance—your height, weight, and physique. When you finish this workout, your physical appearance will command respect immediately; then, as you start mingling and talking to people, your words and actions will exude confidence. This is the biggest advantage you can have over your peers—confidence. Does this workout automatically give you confidence? NO! But it will help you build your confidence, just as it helps you build your strength and stamina.

PREPARING FOR SEAL TRAINING (BUD/S)

The primary goal of this workout program is to prepare and teach individuals about the challenges they will face at Basic Underwater Demolition/SEAL training (BUD/S). The secondary goal is to provide men and women with a progressively difficult 12-week workout that will challenge them every day. If you are a tri-athlete or a hardcore workout animal, you will enjoy this workout. THIS IS NOT A WORKOUT FOR BEGINNERS! You must be in shape long before you attempt this program. These workouts focus on running, swimming, and Physical Training (PT). PT, also known as calisthenics, is comprised of high-repetition, muscle- and stamina-building exercises that will make you leaner and more muscular than you have ever dreamed.

To achieve the primary goal of this workout, you have to be prepared to take the SEAL "Entrance Exam," also known as the SEAL Physical Fitness Test, or PFT. It consists of the following:

500 yard swim using the side or breaststroke	**(10 minute rest)**
Maximum number of Pushups in 2 minutes	**(2 minute rest)**
Maximum number of Situps in 2 minutes	**(2 minute rest)**
Maximum number of Pull-ups	**(10 minute rest)**
1.5 mile run in boots and pants	

This alone is a tough workout! Every fourth week during the 12-week workout, you will take the SEAL PFT in order to check your progress. You may see that your scores do not change the third and fourth time you take the PFT. This is because you are in the toughest weeks of the workout and are actually burned out (if you are doing all the exercises). But do not fear, because during weeks 10-12, a three-week tapering of intensity takes place and you will rebuild your strength and speed. After the twelfth week, start over at Week One and take the SEAL PFT. After your three-week taper, you will see a huge increase in your numbers and a decrease in your times.

The three-week taper is in the workout in order to prevent over-training. If you are supplementing this workout with heavy weight-lifting workouts, longer swims, and runs during the "easy" weeks, you will NOT see the huge gains that a well-rested athlete will experience.

Below are the minimum times needed to pass the SEAL PFT. As you can see, these scores are not that tough to achieve. However, a person who obtains just the minimum scores will not have a chance to get into BUD/S, due to the enormous competition of highly qualified applicants. The competitive scores are the above average scores that I have seen from men who get accepted into BUD/S. The best scores I have seen are from those incredible athletes you will compete with and work with when you are at BUD/S.

	Minimum Scores	Competitive Range	Best Scores I've Seen
Swim (min.)	12:30	7:00-8:30	5.45 sidestroke
Pushups	42	100-120	150
Situps	50	100-120	135
Pull-ups	8	20-30	42
1.5 Mile (min.)	11:30	8:30-10:00	7:45

Though there are no maximum scores for this "Entrance Exam," it is highly recommended that you give your best effort in all areas, in order to be competitive for this highly sought-after course of instruction.

Your number of pull-ups, pushups, and situps will increase after the 12-week workout. Your 1.5-mile-run time will decrease as you train to get your legs and lungs stronger than they have ever been. Your time for the 500-yard sidestroke or breaststroke swim will also decrease due to the large amount of swimming you will do. Detailed pictures and descriptions of the swimming strokes you will use at BUD/S will help you to perfect your technique.

ABOUT BUD/S

Basic Underwater Demolition/SEAL (BUD/S) training is one of the most physically demanding military programs in the world. BUD/S lasts for twenty-six weeks, with each week getting harder and harder. No one graduates from BUD/S without being challenged in some way. It is impossible to meet all the different demands of BUD/S without mentally pushing yourself to succeed. Graduating from BUD/S is possible (thousands have been successful), but ask any SEAL and they will tell you that something personally challenged them to dig deep within and push themselves to succeed. This is why BUD/S is called the "toughest military training in the world."

BUD/S is divided into three phases. Descriptions of each phase are below.

FIRST PHASE (BASIC CONDITIONING)

First Phase lasts for nine weeks. The first four weeks test you in the areas of soft-sand running in boots, swimming with fins in the ocean, and doing more pull-ups, pushups, and flutter kicks than you have ever imagined doing. On the average, a member of your class will quit each day during the first four weeks. The fifth week is known as "Hell Week." During this week, BUD/S students endure 120 hours of continuous training, with minimal sleep (a total of 3-4 hours—for the entire week). Also known as "Motivational Week," this week is designed to be the ultimate test of the student's physical and mental desire to become a SEAL. Typically, fifty percent of your class will quit or be medically discharged by the time Hell Week is over.

WHY DO HELL WEEK?

The experience of Hell Week is what SEALs draw from when situations are cold, dark, and miserable. It proves to all SEALs that the human body can do ten times the amount of work and endure ten times the amount of pain and discomfort than the average human thinks possible. SEALs learn how to remain calm and react properly in hostile situations; how to persevere in the face of adversity; and most importantly, they learn the value of teamwork. The last three weeks of First Phase are spent learning hydrographic reconnaissance and recuperating a little from your 120-hour personal test. Rarely do men quit after Hell Week.

SECOND PHASE (DIVING)

Diving Phase lasts for seven weeks. During this period, physical training continues and the workouts get harder. Students have to run their four-mile runs a minute faster, swim their two-mile swims five minutes faster, and decrease their obstacle course each week of Second Phase. On top of the progressively difficult physical training, the number one priority of Second Phase is teaching students SCUBA (Self Contained Underwater Breathing Apparatus) diving. Students are taught two types of SCUBA: open circuit (compressed air) and closed circuit (100% oxygen rebreather). After Second Phase, students will be basic combat divers, with the physical ability to insert miles from a target and conduct several types of missions. This skill separates SEALs from all other Special Operations Forces.

THIRD PHASE (LAND WARFARE)

Third Phase lasts for nine weeks. Demolitions, reconnaissance, and land warfare are the number-one priorities of this phase; however, this is also the most physically demanding phase of the three. Ten-mile runs, four-mile swims, and hundreds of pushups, pull-ups and situps must be done several times a week. Skills such as land navigation, small arms handling, small-unit tactics, patrolling techniques, rappelling, and military explosives are also mastered. This training is held at San Clemente Island and is classified. You'll have to get there before you learn any more about the highly physical and technical training of BUD/S Third Phase.

RUNNING AT BUD/S

To most BUD/S students, running is the most physically and mentally challenging exercise they will face. It is extremely important to have a strong running base before you arrive at BUD/S. If you do not, you will be one of the majority who become injured during the First Phase, and will have a greater chance of being dropped from the BUD/S program. Running up to four or five times a week at least three months prior to arriving at BUD/S is absolutely necessary. Chapter Five is devoted to teaching the proper techniques of running in the sand and preventing common overuse injuries.

P.T. AT BUD/S

Upper body strength is a must at BUD/S. BUD/S PT lasts at least two hours and is conducted 3-4 times a week. These workouts can test even the seasoned athlete. TRUST ME; DON'T GO TO BUD/S IF YOU HAVE NEVER DONE THE EXERCISES IN THIS BOOK! You should be able to do several hundred pushups, situps, and flutter kicks in a complete workout. Practice these NOW, before you get to BUD/S.

WARNING: Some of these exercises (flutter kicks, leg levers, abdominal stretches...) have been proven and disproven in certain studies to be harmful to your lower back. Navy SEALs have been performing these exercises for over 30 years. Former SEALs in their fifties and sixties still perform these exercises—but do these exercises at your own risk!

SWIMMING AT BUD/S

You will have two-mile timed ocean swims wearing fins every week at BUD/S. It is an absolute necessity to swim with fins prior to arriving at BUD/S. You have to strengthen your ankles and hip flexors by swimming with fins. There is no other way to prepare yourself, and the swimming will be extra challenging for you if you are not prepared. However, the biggest challenge to all BUD/S students is the water temperature—70 degrees in the summer, 55 degrees in the winter. It does not take long to become hypothermic in temperatures this cold. Ask any SEAL and he will tell you that getting used to being cold was the hardest part of BUD/S. Most of the students who quit say they do so because the water was too cold for them.

BUD/S OBSTACLE COURSE

The BUD/S "O-Course" is a test of upper body strength and cardiovascular stamina. The only way to improve at the O-Course is by constantly practicing. It will help if you climb ropes and do hundreds of pull-ups prior to arriving at BUD/S. Obstacles with ropes surrounded by soft sand will challenge anyone, but it will break a person who has slacked off on his upper body exercises. Climb ropes as often as you run—four to five times per week!

FINAL COMMENTS ABOUT BUD/S

BUD/S is said to be the "toughest military training in the world." It is definitely challenging both mentally and physically. The instructors at BUD/S will make demands on your body for six months. You must be in the best shape of your life to succeed at BUD/S; but more importantly, you must be mentally focused and strong or you will become one of the 70-75% who drop out of training. The workout I designed will make you physically fit. If you have the desire to stick to this workout every day, by the end you might just have what it takes to succeed at BUD/S. You will definitely be physically prepared, but will you be mentally prepared? That is up to you.

This is what you must prepare yourself for:

First Phase	Second Phase	Third Phase
four-mile timed runs	four-mile timed runs	four-mile timed runs
up to one-mile swims	up to two-mile ocean swims	up to three-mile ocean swims
obstacle courses	obstacle courses	obstacle courses
50m underwater swim	5.5-mile ocean swim*	15-mile timed run*
upper body PT	upper body PT	upper body PT
soft-sand runs	soft-sand runs	soft-sand runs
HELLWEEK*		

*Special one-time events. All other events occur WEEKLY!

HOW DO YOU MENTALLY PREPARE YOURSELF FOR BUD/S?

First, being physically prepared will help you become mentally tough. Just as your endurance will grow each day with this program, so will your confidence. Knowing in your heart that you can complete the evolutions listed above without even thinking of quitting is the secret to excelling at BUD/S. For me, knowing that if I quit, I had to serve on a ship for the next five years was enough motivation. Others have something to prove to themselves, their family, or their friends. The key is to find what motivates you to succeed and then stay focused on that motivator when the days are long and the nights are just beginning. During Hell Week, take one hour at a time. Do not think that because you are exhausted and are only two hours into the 120-hour week that you cannot complete Hell Week. Instead think about making it to the next meal. Students get to sit, rest, and eat for almost an hour every six hours during Hell Week.

COLD WATER

It will help if you become accustomed to ocean water, especially water temperature in the 60s. Ocean swims and body surfing are great ways to prepare yourself for the "Surf Zone." If you do not have access to ocean water, swim with fins in a pool for a couple of hours a few times a week. You have to realize that the BUD/S instructors can only keep you in the water for a certain period of time—NOTHING WILL LAST FOREVER.

SAFETY!

I do not recommend swimming alone in a pool, but especially not in the ocean. Navy SEALs always have a "swim buddy" with them no mater what they are doing. If you do not have a friend who shares your same desires and work ethic, at least have a lifeguard watch you swim.

Good luck—I hope you find what motivates you to never quit!

EQUIPMENT AND FACILITIES NEEDED FOR THIS WORKOUT:

- Access to a pool, either 25m or 25 yd, 50m or 50 yd.

- Access to a track or measured running area, 400m/400 yd.

- Access to pull-up bars and dip bars (parallel bars).

STRETCHING

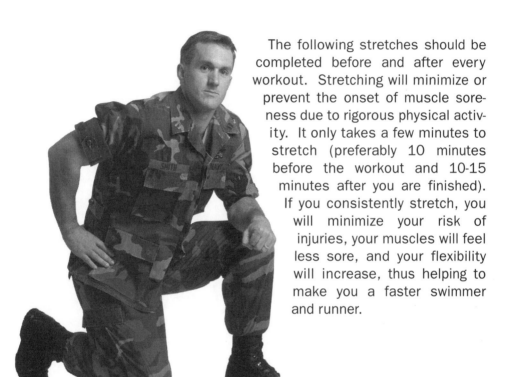

The following stretches should be completed before and after every workout. Stretching will minimize or prevent the onset of muscle soreness due to rigorous physical activity. It only takes a few minutes to stretch (preferably 10 minutes before the workout and 10-15 minutes after you are finished). If you consistently stretch, you will minimize your risk of injuries, your muscles will feel less sore, and your flexibility will increase, thus helping to make you a faster swimmer and runner.

PRE/POST WORKOUT STRETCHING ROUTINE

Stretches	Repetitions/Time:
Jog	1/4 mile
Neck rotations	30 sec.
Arm and Shoulder	30 sec. each arm
Arm Circles	1 min.
Chest	30 sec.
Abdominal	30 sec.
Lower Back	30 sec.
Groin Stretch	30 sec.
ITB	30 sec. each leg
Thighs	30 sec. each leg.
Toe Touches	30 sec.
Calves	30 sec. each leg
Hamstring	30 sec.
Jumping Jacks	25 (4-count)

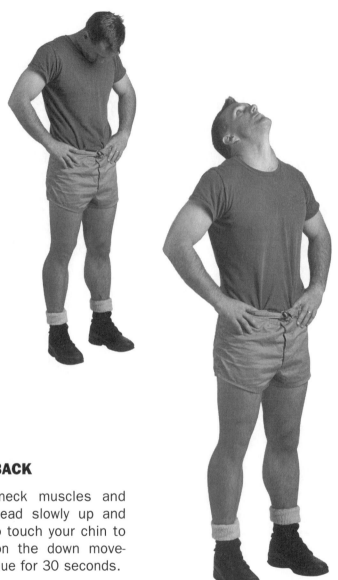

FRONT TO BACK

Relax your neck muscles and move your head slowly up and down. Try to touch your chin to your chest on the down movement. Continue for 30 seconds.

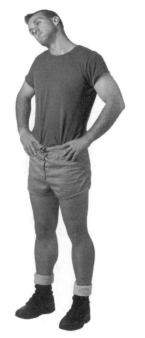

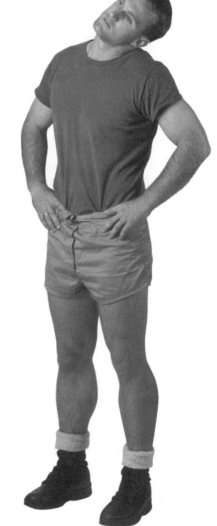

SIDE TO SIDE

Relax your neck muscles and move your head slowly to the left and right. Move your head as if you were trying to touch your shoulder to your ear. Continue for 30 seconds.

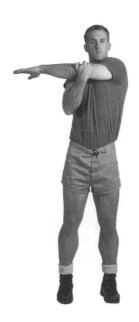

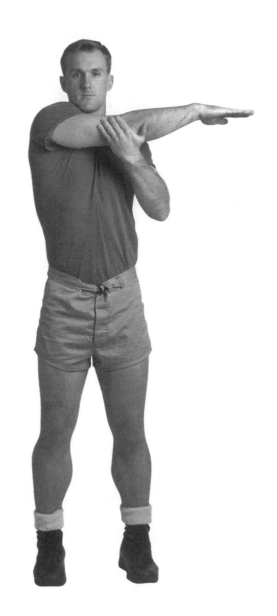

ARM AND SHOULDER STRETCH #1

With your left hand, grab your fight arm at the elbow and pull across your body. Hold for 15 seconds—switch arms.

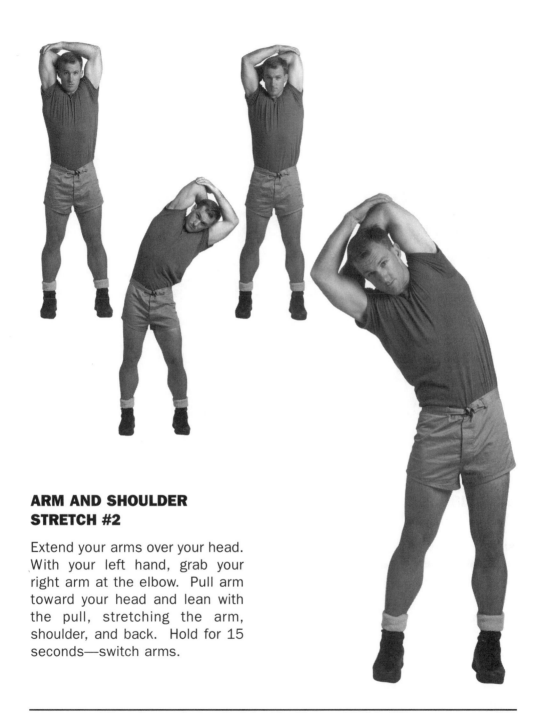

ARM AND SHOULDER STRETCH #2

Extend your arms over your head. With your left hand, grab your right arm at the elbow. Pull arm toward your head and lean with the pull, stretching the arm, shoulder, and back. Hold for 15 seconds—switch arms.

Arm Circles

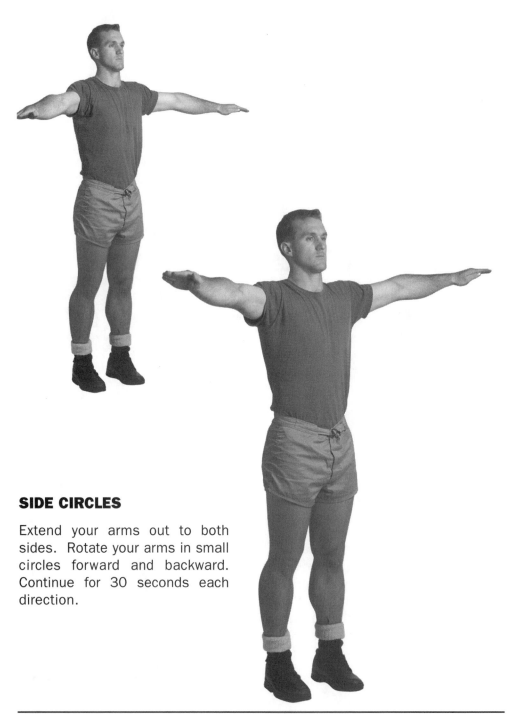

SIDE CIRCLES

Extend your arms out to both sides. Rotate your arms in small circles forward and backward. Continue for 30 seconds each direction.

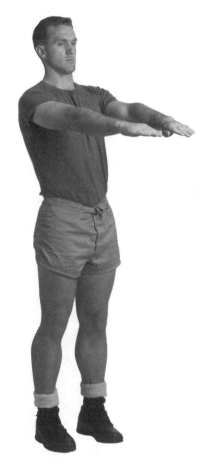

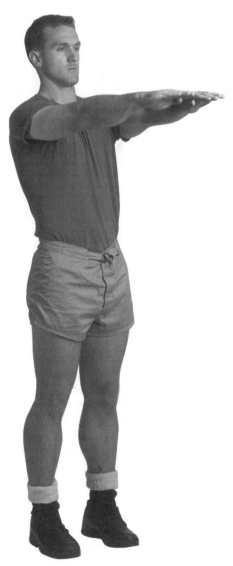

FRONT CIRCLES

Extend both arms in front of you.
Rotate your arms in small circles
inward and outward.   Continue
for 30 seconds each direction.

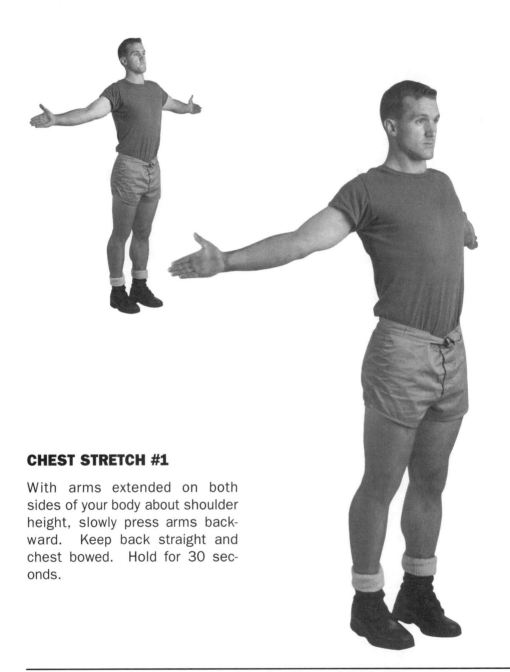

CHEST STRETCH #1

With arms extended on both sides of your body about shoulder height, slowly press arms backward. Keep back straight and chest bowed. Hold for 30 seconds.

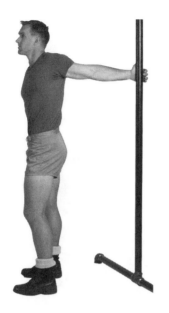

WALL STRETCH

Place right arm on wall about shoulder height. Turn body away from the wall to the left. Hold arm in place. Hold for 15 seconds. Switch and repeat.

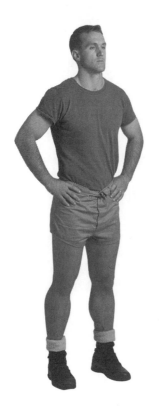

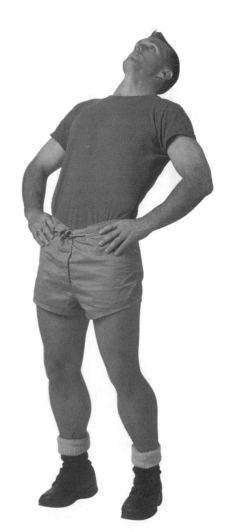

STANDING

With your hands on your waist, slowly lean backward by pushing your hips forward and slightly arching your back. Hold for 15 seconds—repeat.

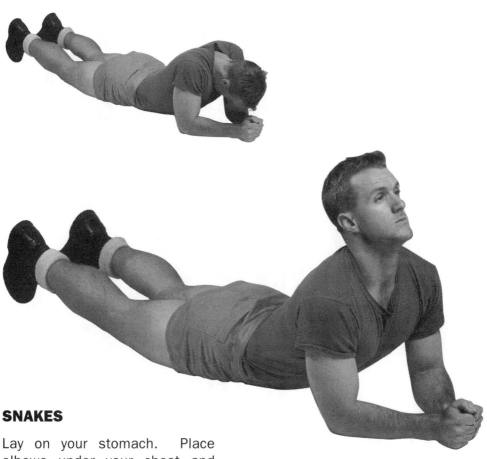

SNAKES

Lay on your stomach. Place elbows under your chest and slowly lift your head and shoulders up, stretching your abdominal muscles. Hold for 15 seconds—repeat.

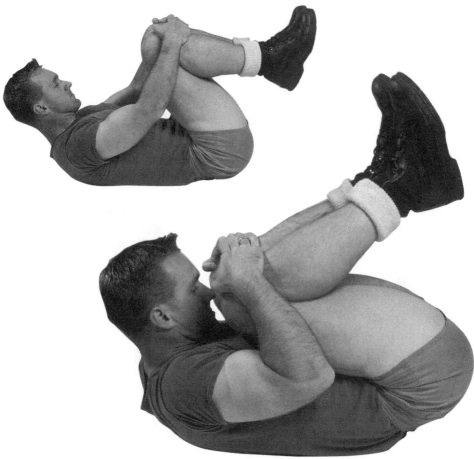

CHEST TO KNEES

Lay on your back. Bring your knees to your chest and your head toward your knees. Hold for 15 seconds.

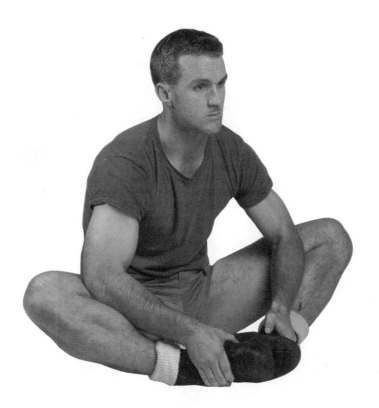

BUTTERFLY

Sit on the floor with both legs bent outward and the soles of your feet touching each other. Grab your ankles with your hands and push down on your thighs with your elbows. Hold for 15 seconds—repeat.

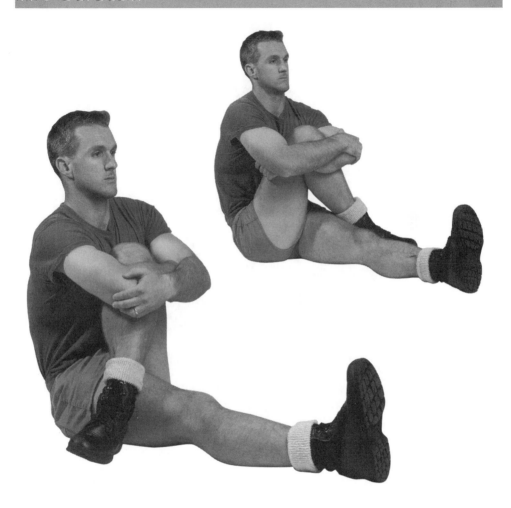

ITB STRETCH #1 (ILIO TIBIAL BAND)

Sit on the floor with both legs extended in front of you. Cross your right leg over your left. Bend and pull right leg to your chest and hold for 15 seconds. Switch and repeat.*

*Author's Note: Injury to the ITB due to overuse is very common among BUD/S students. For this reason, injury to the ITB is sometimes referred to as "I Tried BUD/S."

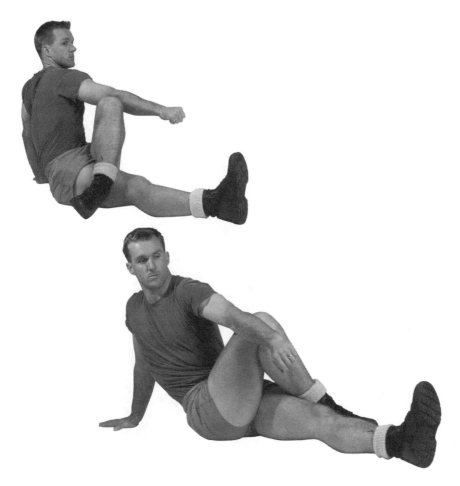

ITB STRETCH #2

In the same position as Stretch #1, twist to the side of bent leg to stretch your lower back and ITB. Try to look in the opposite direction of your feet. Hold for 15 seconds. Switch and repeat.

Thigh Stretches

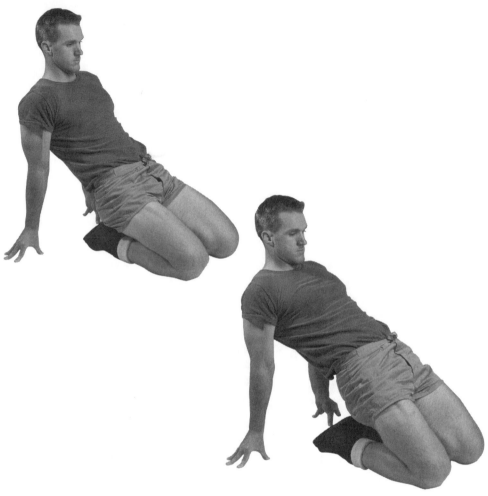

SITTING

Sit on your knees and heels. Lean backward so you can touch the floor behind you. Push your hips upward and hold for 15 seconds—repeat.

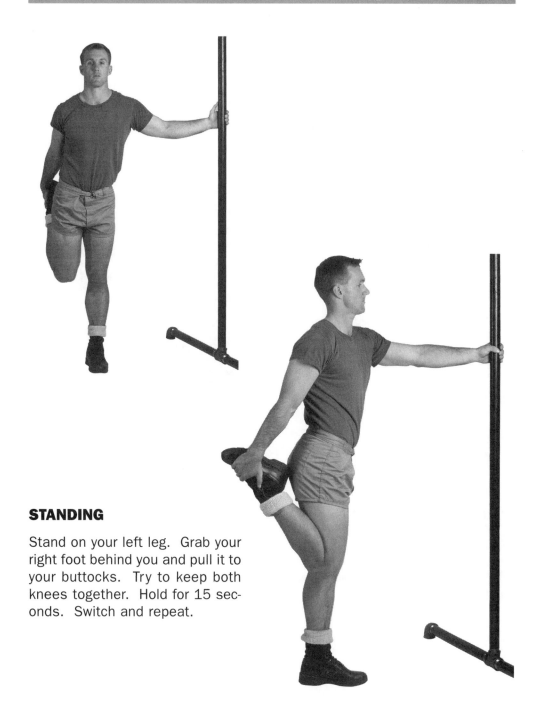

STANDING

Stand on your left leg. Grab your right foot behind you and pull it to your buttocks. Try to keep both knees together. Hold for 15 seconds. Switch and repeat.

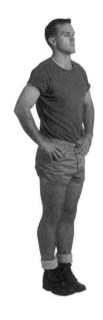

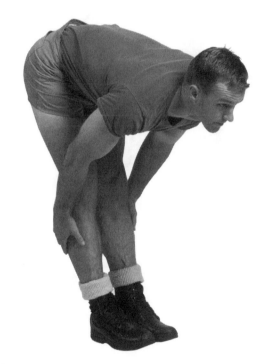

STANDING OR SITTING

With your feet together, bend at
the waist and grab the back of
your calves with both hands.
Hold for 15 seconds—repeat.

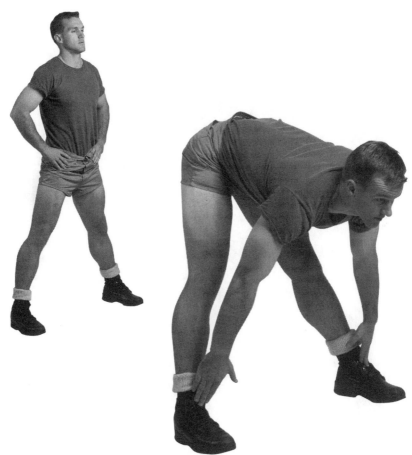

STANDING OR SITTING

With feet spread apart, bend at
the waist and hold your back flat,
stretching your hamstrings and
lower back. Hold for 15 seconds—repeat.

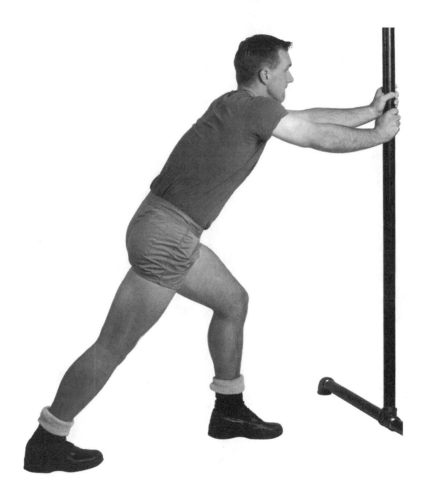

GASTROCNEMIUS

Stand about four feet away from a wall or other sturdy object. With most of your weight on one leg, keep that leg straight and lean into the wall. Hold for 15 seconds—switch legs and repeat.

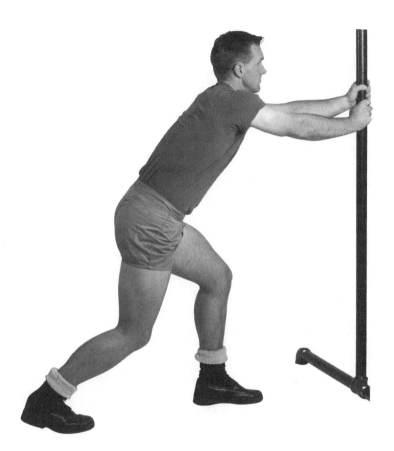

SOLEUS

Same stance as the Gastrocnemius Stretch, but bend your back knee slightly. You will feel the stretch in your Achilles tendon. Hold for 15 seconds—switch and repeat.

Hamstring Stretch

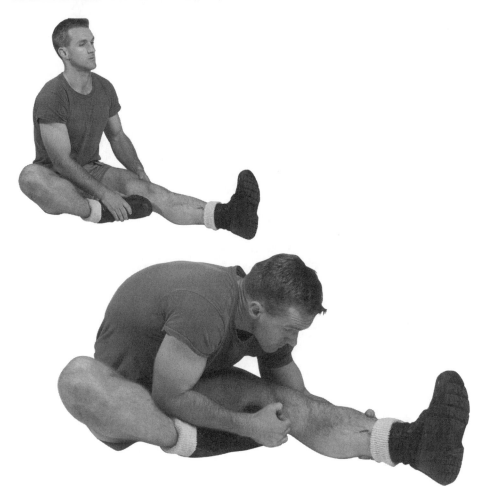

HURDLER STRIDE

Sit on the floor with legs extended in front of you. Bend right knee and place the sole of your right foot against the inside of your left knee. Grab feet and hold stretch for 15 seconds. Switch and repeat.

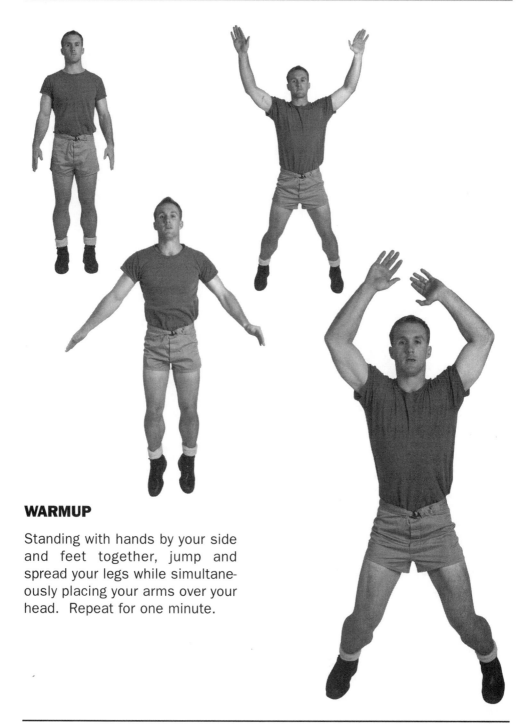

WARMUP

Standing with hands by your side and feet together, jump and spread your legs while simultaneously placing your arms over your head. Repeat for one minute.

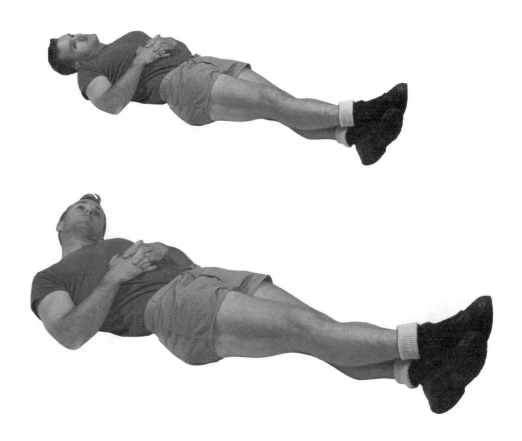

NECK EXERCISE #1: SIDE TO SIDE

Lay on your back. Lift your head off the floor and move it from side to side for specified number of repetitions.*

*Author's Note: The number of repetitions for each exercise will vary depending on which day of which week of the program you are completing (see the 12 Weeks to BUD/S Workout chapter beginning on page 111). For example, in Week One, you will do 20 repetitions of the side-to-side neck exercise shown above. In Week Ten, you will do 100 repetitions of this exercise.

Physical Training, or PT, is a series of calisthenics and other exercises which are designed to strengthen your body. A combination of these exercises is referred to as "grinder PT" at BUD/S.

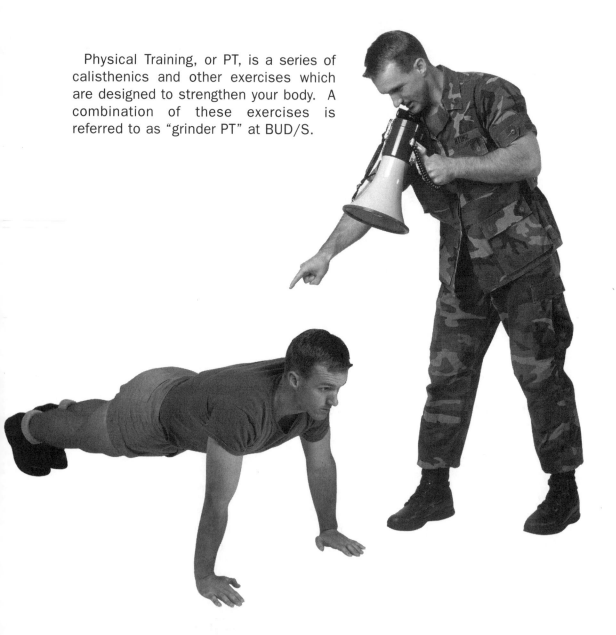

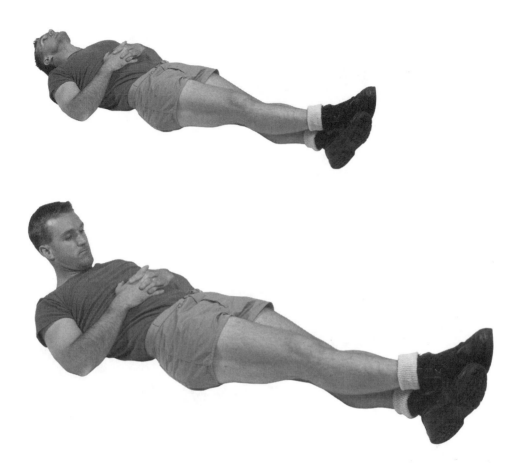

NECK EXERCISE #2: UP AND DOWN

Lay on your back. Lift your head off the floor and move it up and down for specified number of repetitions.

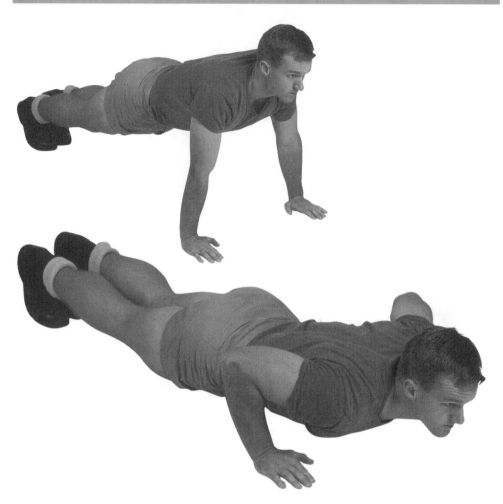

PUSHUPS: REGULAR

With hands at shoulder width, place your palms on the ground, keeping your feet together and back straight. Push your body up until your arms are straight. Touch chest to ground each repetition.

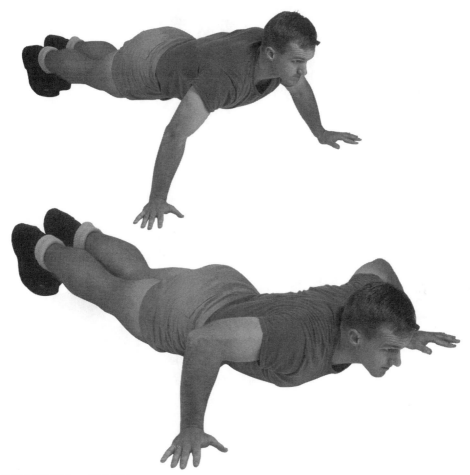

PUSHUPS: WIDE

With hands wider than shoulder width, place your palms on the ground, keeping feet together and back straight. Push your body up until your arms are straight. Touch chest to ground each repetition.

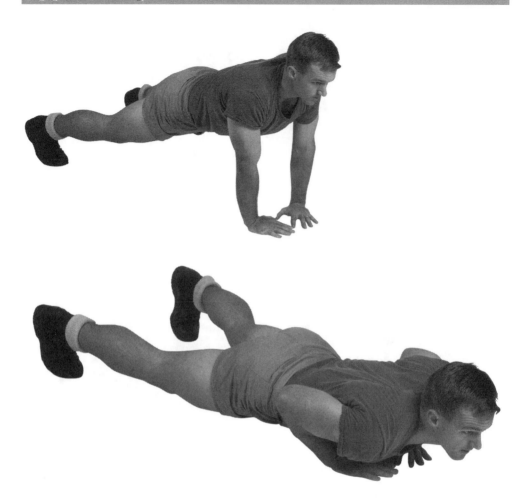

PUSHUPS: TRICEPS

With hands touching, forming a triangle with your index fingers and thumbs meeting (as shown above), place palms on the ground, spreading your legs and keeping your back straight. Push your body up until your arms are straight. Touch chest to hands each repetition.

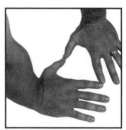

DETAIL

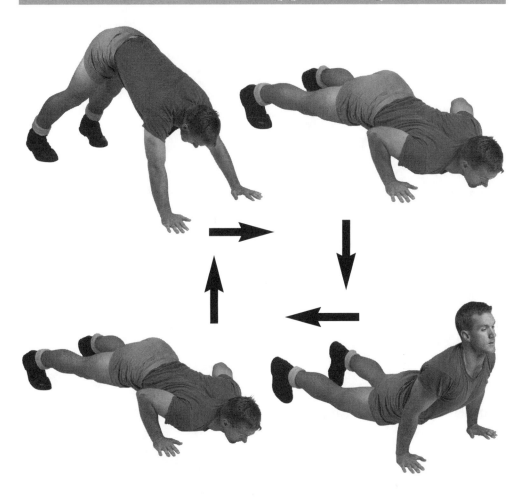

PUSHUPS: DIVE BOMBERS

Get into the pushup position, but bend at the waist and stick your buttocks in the air (Figure 1). Keeping your buttocks in the air, place chest to the ground in between your hands (Figure 2). Continue forward movement and push your chest through your hands and up by straightening your arms (Figure 3). Reverse the process and return back to starting position (Figure 4).

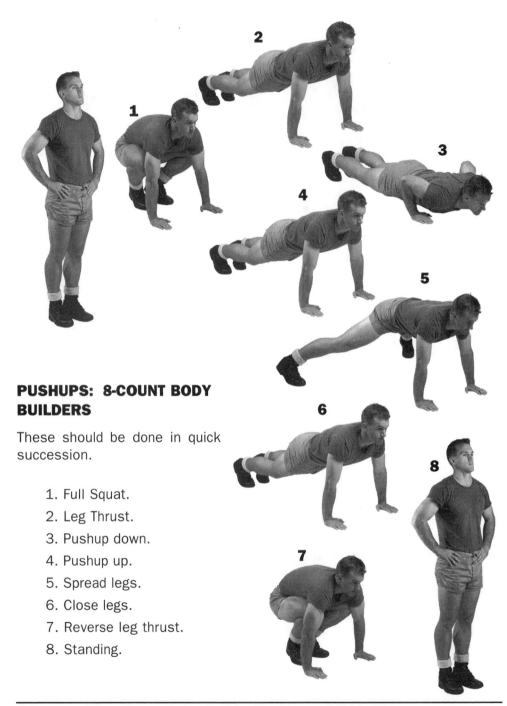

PUSHUPS: 8-COUNT BODY BUILDERS

These should be done in quick succession.

1. Full Squat.
2. Leg Thrust.
3. Pushup down.
4. Pushup up.
5. Spread legs.
6. Close legs.
7. Reverse leg thrust.
8. Standing.

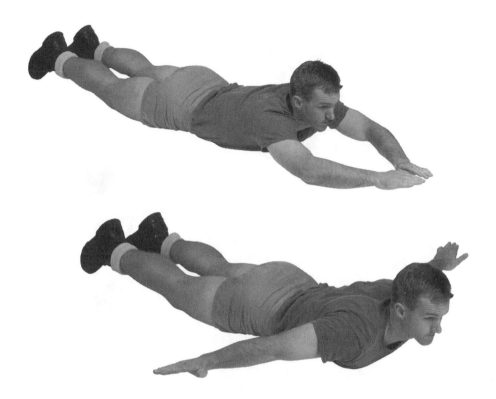

ARM HAULERS

Lay on your stomach with your back arched slightly. Move your arms from the starting position over your head to your side (as if you were swimming). Keep your feet off the ground as well. This exercise works shoulders, lower back, and buttocks.

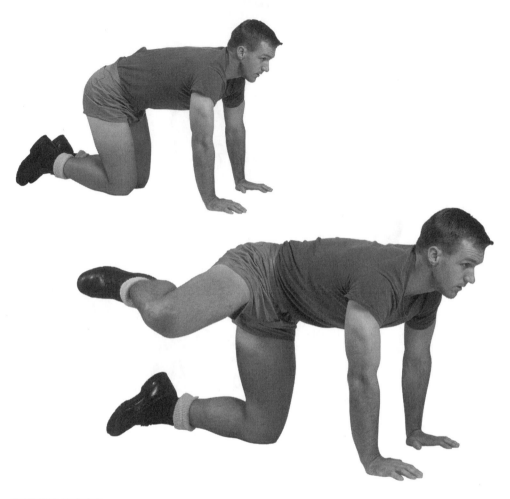

DIRTY DOGS

Get into the "all fours" position. Lift your leg from your hip joint to the side for the specified number of repetitions. You may drop to your elbows for more comfort on your lower back. Switch sides and repeat.

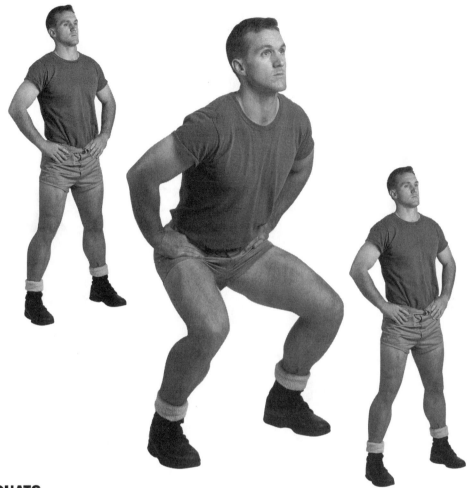

SQUATS

With feet about shoulder width apart, back straight, and eyes looking up, lower yourself by bending your legs almost 90 degrees at the knees. Slowly raise yourself after you have reached almost 90 degrees.

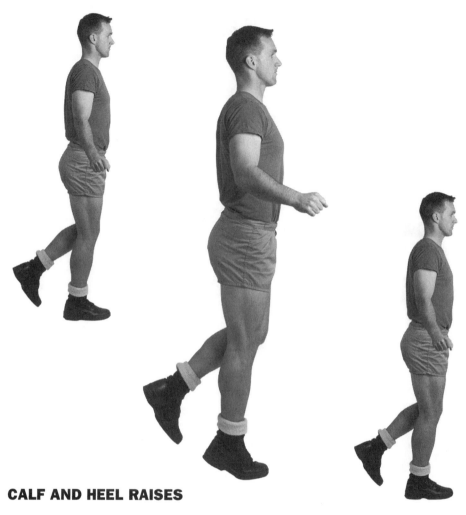

CALF AND HEEL RAISES

Stand on one leg. Lift yourself up onto the balls of your feet by flexing the ankle joint and calf muscle. Switch legs and repeat for specified number of repetitions.

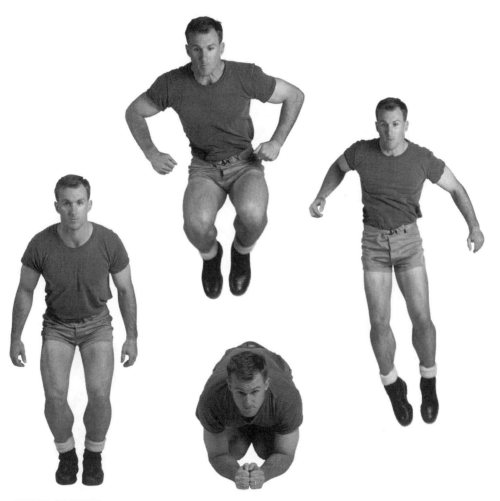

JUMPOVERS

Stand next to an object approximately 1.5-2 feet high. Jump from one side to the other for specified number of repetitions. Try to hit the ground on one side and jump back immediately after touching. Try not to double bounce.

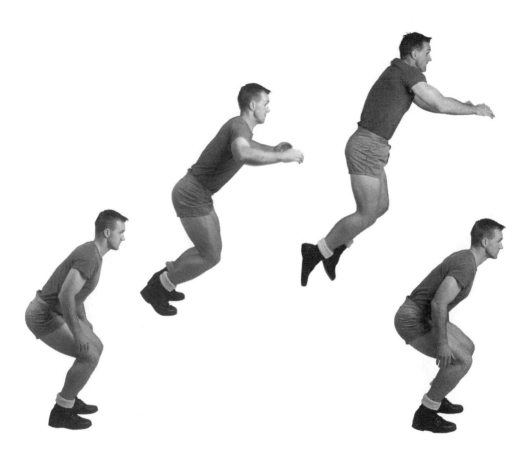

FROG HOPS

From the squatting position, jump forward as far as you can. Repeat for specified number of repetitions.

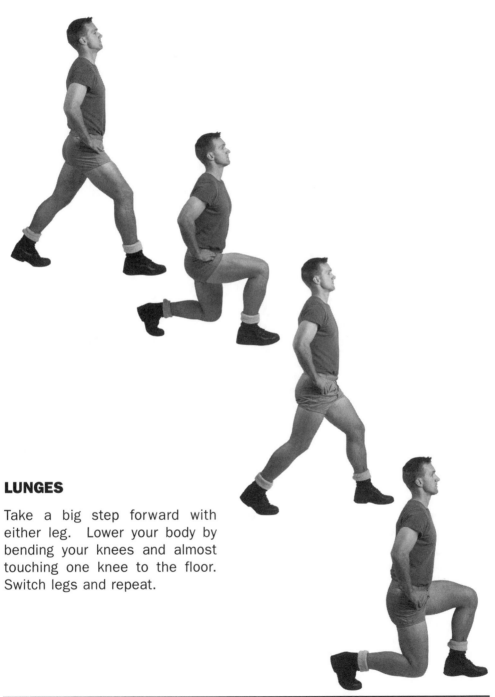

LUNGES

Take a big step forward with either leg. Lower your body by bending your knees and almost touching one knee to the floor. Switch legs and repeat.

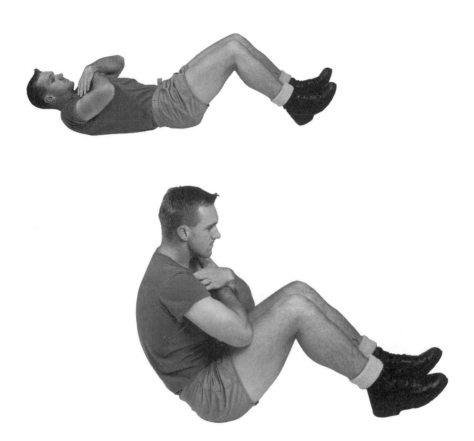

SITUPS: REGULAR

Lay on your back with your arms crossed over your chest and your knees slightly bent. Raise your upper body off the floor by contracting your stomach muscles. Touch your elbows to your thighs and repeat. Make sure you touch your shoulder blades to the floor each time.

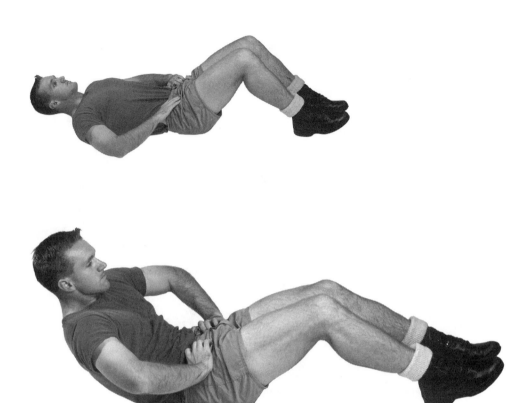

1/2 SITUP

Lay on your back and place your hands on your hips. Lift your upper body so your lower back just comes off the floor, then slowly let yourself back down to the starting position. Repeat for specified number of repetitions.

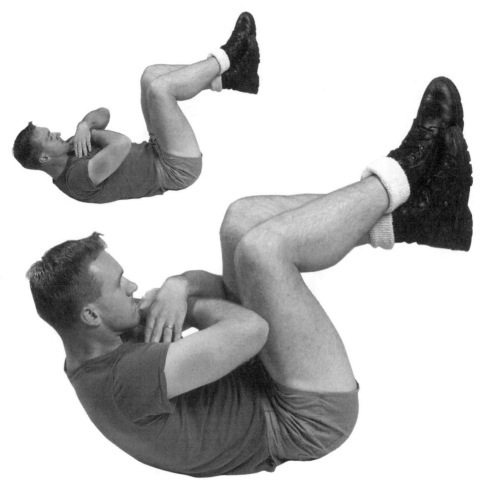

CRUNCHES: REGULAR

Lay on your back with your legs up in the air and bent at the knees, forming a 90 degree angle with your legs. Bring your elbows to your knees. DO NOT PUT YOUR HANDS BEHIND YOUR HEAD AND PULL ON YOUR NECK.

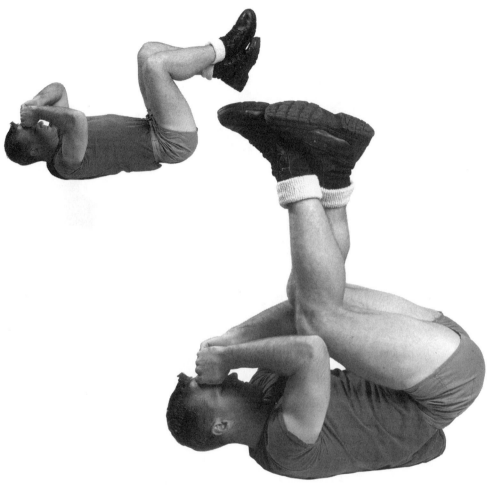

CRUNCHES: REVERSE

Lay on your back with your legs up in the air and bent at the knees, forming a 90 degree angle with your legs. Bring your knees to your elbows, lifting your lower back and buttocks off the ground. Keep your upper body still.

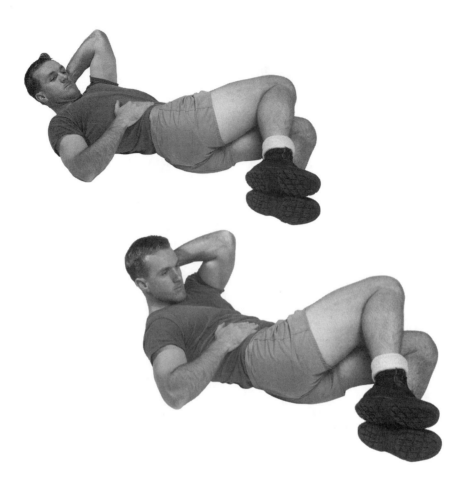

CRUNCHES: RIGHT

Lay with your shoulders and back flat on the floor, twisting your waist and legs so that you are laying on the left side of your hip. Crunch upward with your left arm and shoulder across your body toward the right side of your hip.

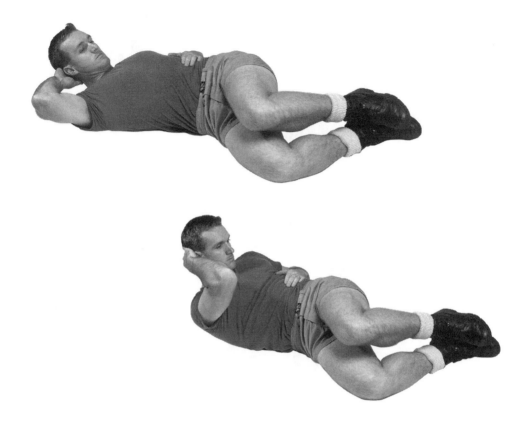

CRUNCHES: LEFT

Lay with your shoulders and back flat on the floor, twisting your waist and legs so that you are laying on the right side of your hip. Crunch upward with your right arm and shoulder across your body toward the left side of your hip.

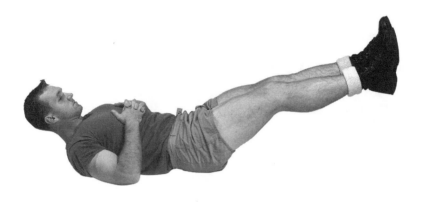

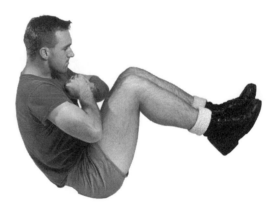

SITUPS: ATOMIC

Lay on your back. Lift your feet 6 inches off the floor and pull your knees toward your chest while simultaneously lifting your upper body off the floor.

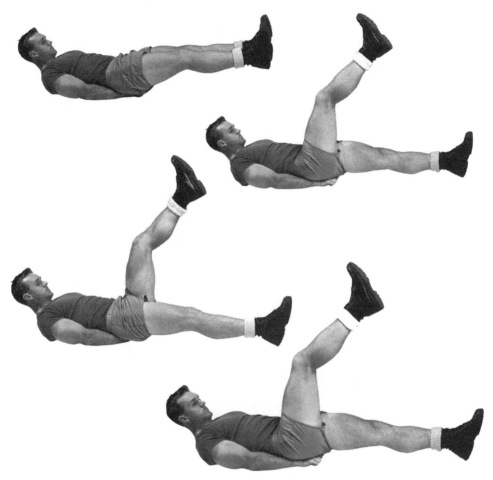

4-COUNT FLUTTER KICKS

Place your hands under your hips. Lift legs 6 inches off the ground and begin "walking," raising each leg approximately 3 feet off the ground. Keep your legs straight and constantly moving. With each "step" you take, count 1, so the sequence will go as follows: 1, 2, 3, 1; 1, 2, 3, 2; 1, 2, 3, 3; . . . for the specified number of repetitions.

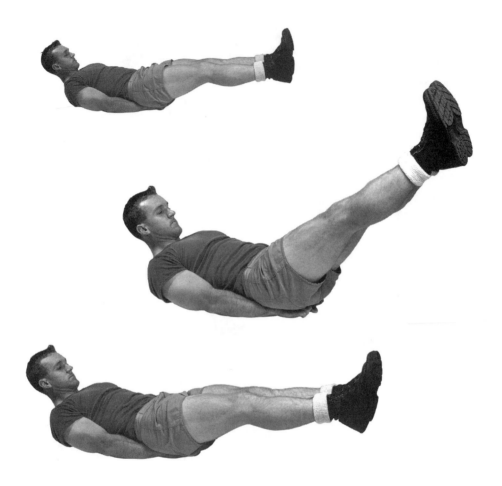

LEG LEVERS

Lay on your back with your hands under your hips and your legs together 6 inches off the floor. Lift your legs about 3 feet off the floor and slowly bring them down. Repeat. Do not let your legs touch the ground.

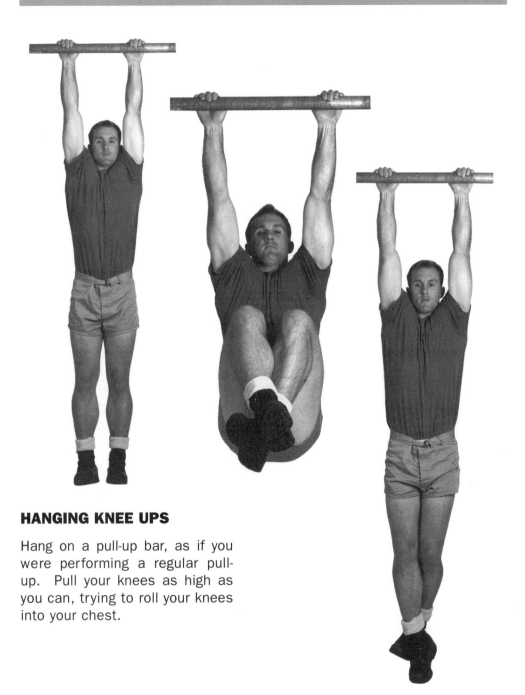

HANGING KNEE UPS

Hang on a pull-up bar, as if you were performing a regular pull-up. Pull your knees as high as you can, trying to roll your knees into your chest.

PULL-UPS AND DIPS

There are five different types of pull-ups which work various groups of arm and back muscles. The pull-up workout that requires sets of 2, 4, 6, 8, and 10 repetitions for every type of pull-up is challenging, but offers moments of recovery and rest.

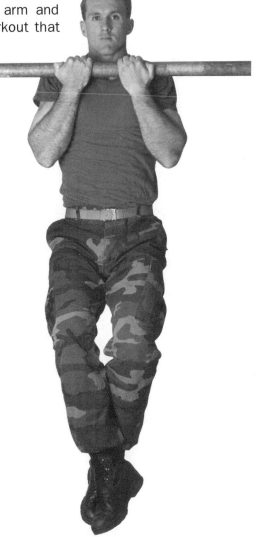

A Word About Pull-ups

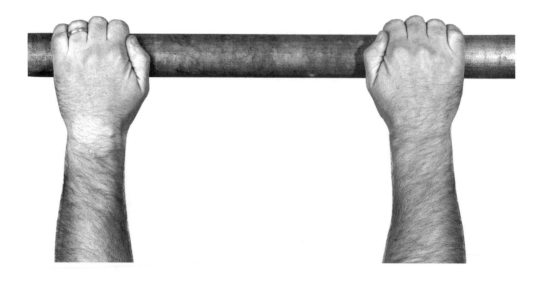

CORRECT GRIP

To strengthen your grip when doing pull-ups, make sure you use the correct grip shown above. This will increase the number of pull-ups you can do. Place your thumb next to your index finger and grip the bar with your fingers. Do not wrap your thumb around the bar.

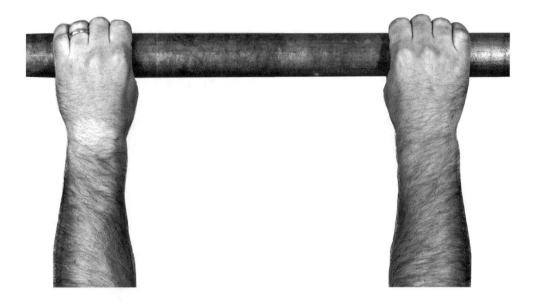

INCORRECT GRIP

The above photo, with thumbs and fingers wrapped around the bar, shows the grip that you should not use when doing pull-ups. With your thumb wrapped around the bar, your grip will weaken more quickly than if you use the proper grip shown on the opposite page.

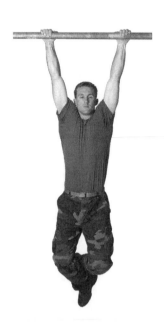

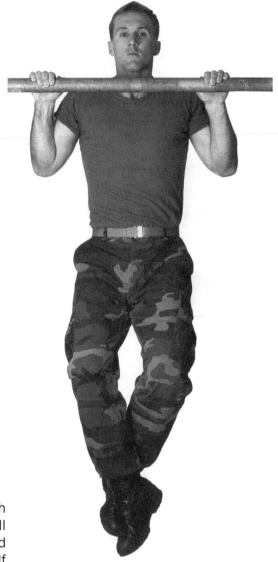

REGULAR GRIP

With hands at shoulder width (see below), grab the bar and pull yourself up so your chin is lifted above the bar. Hold yourself above the bar for one second and let yourself down in a slow, controlled manner.

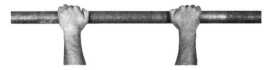

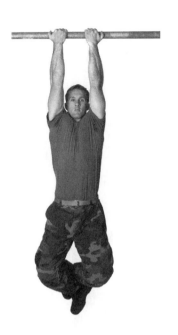

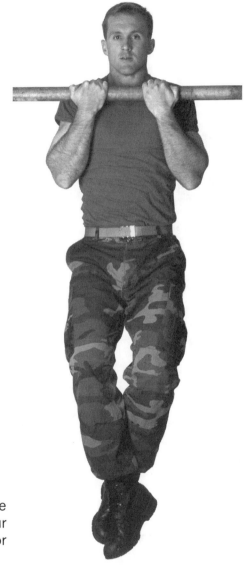

REVERSE GRIP

With your palms facing you (see below), grab the bar and pull your chin over the bar. Repeat for specified number of repetitions.

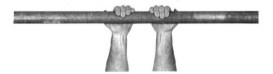

Pull-ups

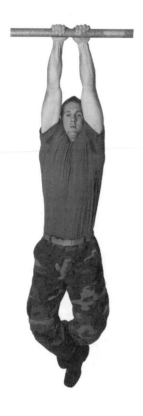

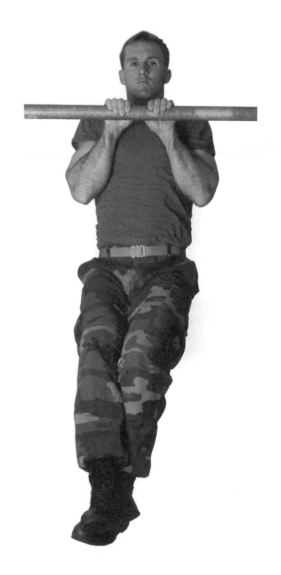

CLOSE GRIP

With your hands touching (or within 1 inch of each other), and palms facing away from you (see below), grab the bar and pull your chin over the bar. Repeat for specified number of repetitions.

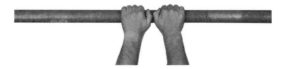

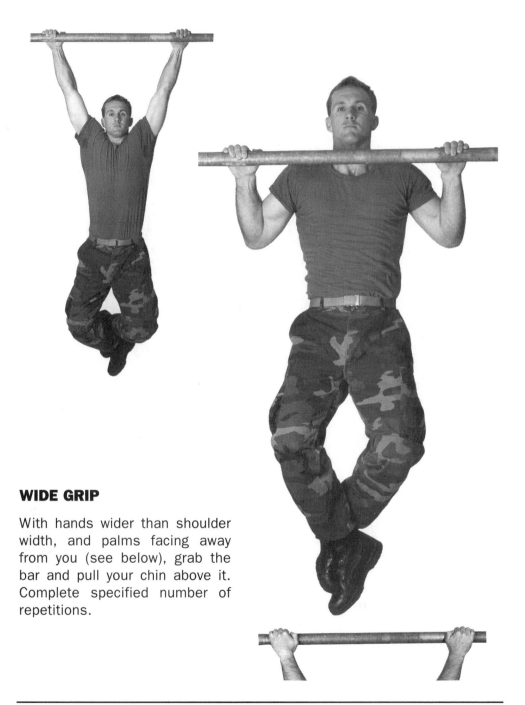

WIDE GRIP

With hands wider than shoulder width, and palms facing away from you (see below), grab the bar and pull your chin above it. Complete specified number of repetitions.

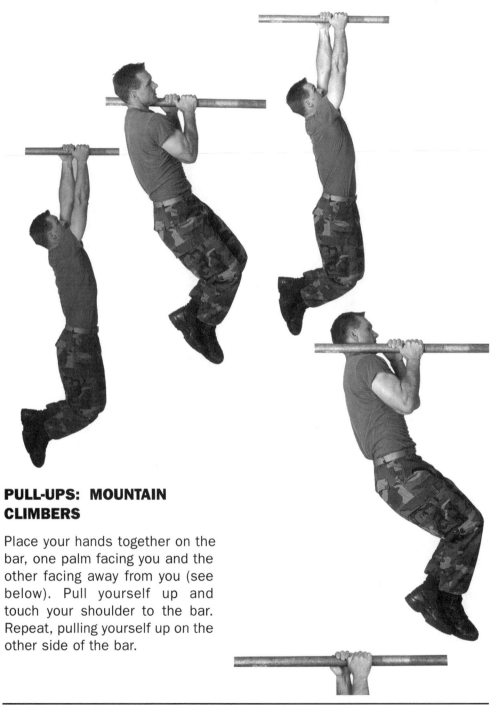

PULL-UPS: MOUNTAIN CLIMBERS

Place your hands together on the bar, one palm facing you and the other facing away from you (see below). Pull yourself up and touch your shoulder to the bar. Repeat, pulling yourself up on the other side of the bar.

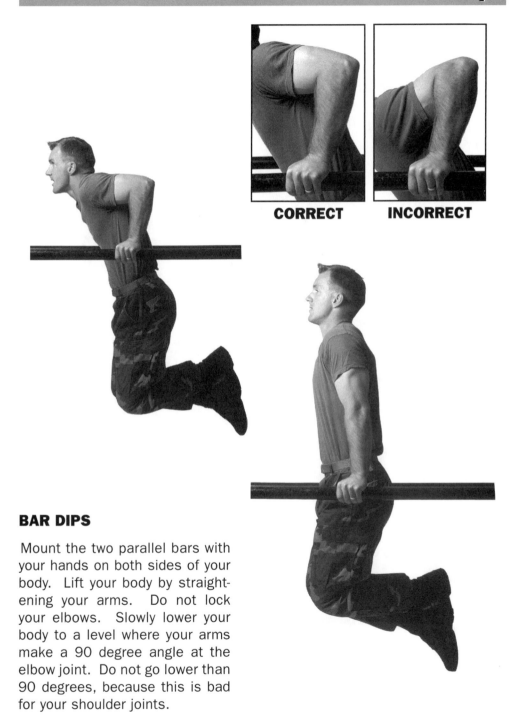

CORRECT   **INCORRECT**

BAR DIPS

Mount the two parallel bars with your hands on both sides of your body. Lift your body by straightening your arms. Do not lock your elbows. Slowly lower your body to a level where your arms make a 90 degree angle at the elbow joint. Do not go lower than 90 degrees, because this is bad for your shoulder joints.

RUNNING
AT BUD/S

Running in sand is more difficult than running on pavement, but less stressful on your joints. After several weeks of running in sand, your leg muscles will become stronger and you will have more stamina than ever before. Running is also an excellent cross-training tool to increase leg muscle definition, especially when you sprint regularly.

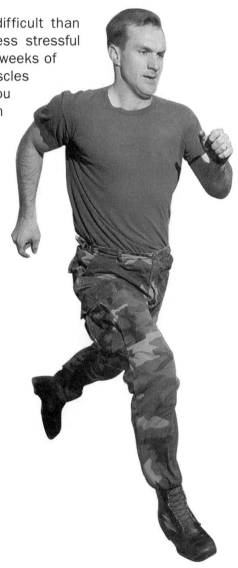

There is nothing quite like running in soft sand at BUD/S to challenge your desire to "never quit." It definitely helps to run on the beach prior to reporting to BUD/S because you'll need time to learn the techniques and adjust to the leg fatigue associated with soft-sand running.

To pass these runs, all you have to do is **stay with the pack**. Do not fall behind or you will be further tested through the formation of the GOON SQUAD. The GOON SQUAD is the group that does not stay with the pack on the platoon runs. If by the end of a run a student is not back in formation, they will receive extra physical training in order to "motivate" them. A weekly four-mile timed run on the beach wearing combat boots is a test that will challenge even the best runners. Here are some training tips that will help you decrease your run times and stay with the pack.

RUNNING ON SOFT SAND AND PAVEMENT

When running in the soft sand at BUD/S, stepping in footprints or previously made depressions is the biggest key to success. In soft-sand running, it is essential to change your stride to more of a shuffle and dig your toes into the sand. This will work your calves more than normal pavement running.

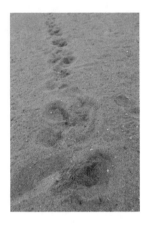

On pavement or hard-packed sand, **heel-toe contact** will help you with opening your stride and decreasing the stress on your knees and hips. Your foot should strike the pavement or hard surface with the heel of your foot and should roll forward across the ball and push off the ground with your toes.

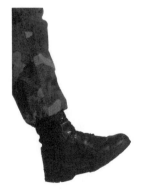
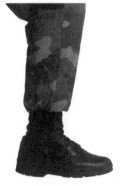
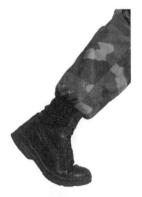

A good way to check your stride is the audible test. If you can hear your feet hit the ground, you are probably running flat-footed and need to open your stride. Shin splints and stress fractures soon accompany this unnatural style of running. So—run quietly!

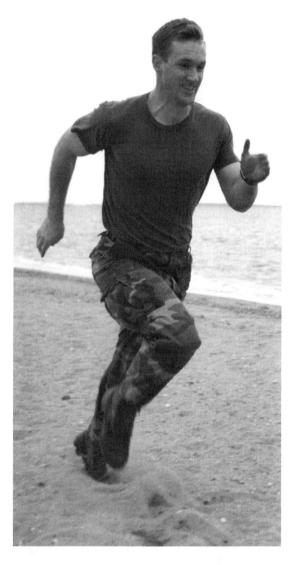

Regardless of the running surface, by far the most important technique of proper running is **breathing**. The proper breath is a very deep inhalation and exhalation. It should feel like a yawn. People who tend to take rapid, shallow breaths create carbon-dioxide build-up, increase their heart rate, and will encourage muscle cramps. Deep breaths get more oxygen to your muscles, rid your body of carbon dioxide, and aid in reducing fatigue.

Relaxing the upper body is another important running technique. When you are running, the only body parts that should be working are your lungs and your legs. If your upper body, fists, or face are clenched or flexed while running, the blood that should be going to your legs is sent to the flexed body parts as well, thus decreasing the amount of oxygen to your legs. Try to relax and breathe deeply.

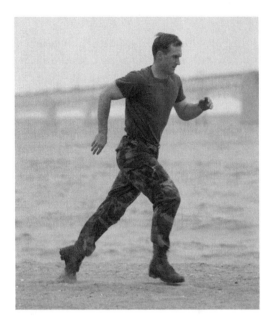

A full arm swing will help you get into a good running step and breathing rhythm. Your hands should swing in a straight line from your hips to your chest. Elbows should be bent slightly and hands should be loose and unclenched.

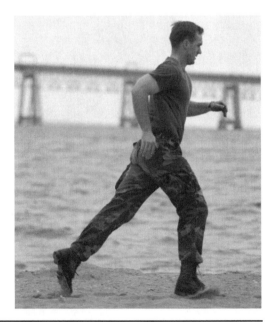

SWIMMING AT BUD/S

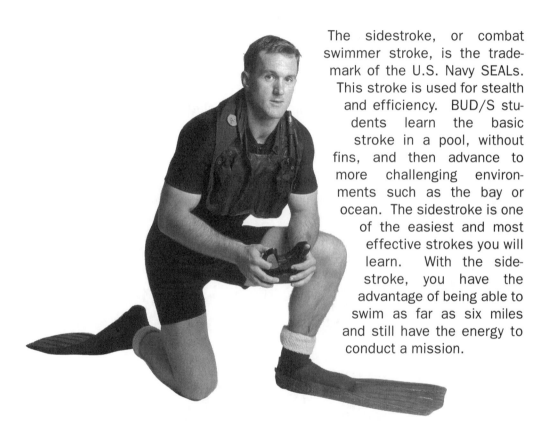

The sidestroke, or combat swimmer stroke, is the trademark of the U.S. Navy SEALs. This stroke is used for stealth and efficiency. BUD/S students learn the basic stroke in a pool, without fins, and then advance to more challenging environments such as the bay or ocean. The sidestroke is one of the easiest and most effective strokes you will learn. With the sidestroke, you have the advantage of being able to swim as far as six miles and still have the energy to conduct a mission.

SIDESTROKE WITHOUT FINS

Swimming sidestroke without fins requires timing and coordination of kicks, arm pulls, and breathing. Preparing for the SEAL PFT 500-yard swim test will be easier if you follow the techniques and recommendations below:

1. **Kick off the wall.** Every length of the pool, turn around, inhale, and kick off the wall, gliding until momentum almost stops. Start exhaling. Then, staying underwater, give one big double-arm pull and glide with your hands by your waist. Angle yourself toward the surface as you glide, because by this time you will need to breathe. When you break the surface to breathe, you should be about 8-10 yards off the wall—with only minimal physical effort!

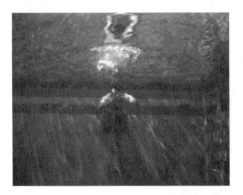 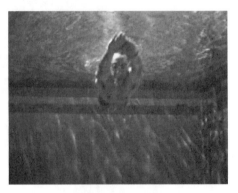

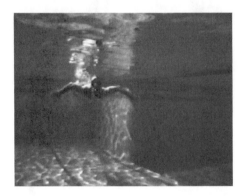

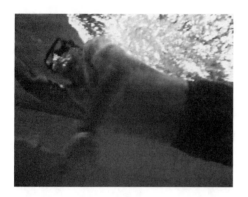
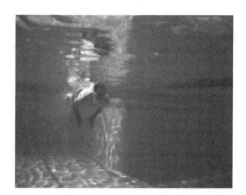

2. **First breath.** Turn to your side and extend your bottom arm over your head. Your top arm remains by your side as you pause for a big inhalation.

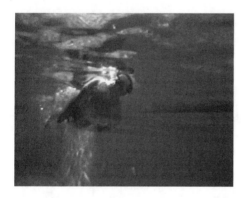
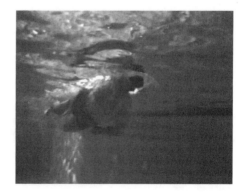

3. **Pull and kick coordination.** As your bottom arm begins its stroke and pulls toward your side (your top arm is already by your side), breathe, then move your arms over your head together. As your arms move forward, your top leg should also move forward as your legs spread to prepare for the big scissor kick.

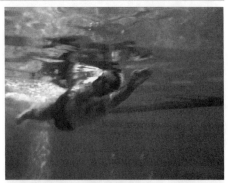

As you pull your top arm back to your side, kick and exhale at the same time. As your legs come together, the top arm should have completed its stroke and be by your side again as the bottom arm stays extended over your head. This is the glide position. Glide and breathe as you begin to pull your bottom arm to your side again.

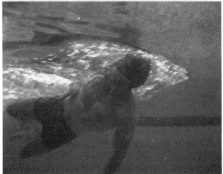

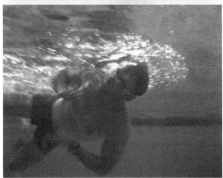

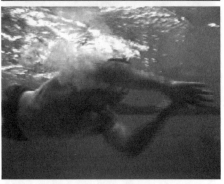

4. **Flutter kick in between scissor kicks.** To help keep your momentum going and your body streamlined in the water, use 6-12" flutter kicks in between the powerful scissor kicks.

SCISSOR KICK   ## FLUTTER KICK

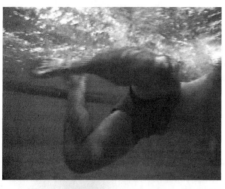 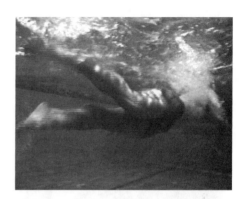

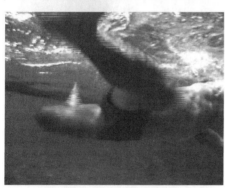 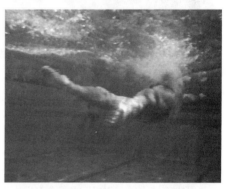

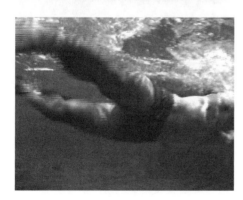 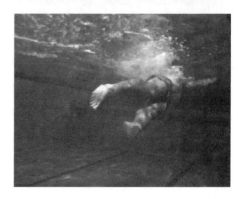

SIDESTROKE WITH FINS

You will use fins 99% of the time once you have entered the First Phase of BUD/S. Your ankles and hip flexors must be strong in order to do this; therefore, I recommend that you are able to swim at least one mile (with fins), without stopping, in less than 30 minutes before arriving at BUD/S. Sidestroke with fins is similar to the sidestroke without fins with only the following differences:

1. **Constant flutter kicks.** With fins on your feet, your biggest source of power will naturally be your legs, so kick constantly in order to be propelled through the water.

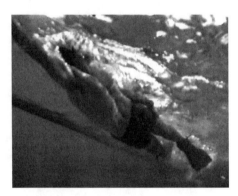

2. **Swimming in a straight line.** About every five to ten strokes, it is important to look forward in order to check if you are swimming in a straight line. This does not need to be done in the swimming pool; however, it is important in the open ocean to have a visual reference when surface swimming to check accuracy.

3. **Arm pull and breathing coordination.** As your top arm completes its stroke and the bottom arm is beginning to pull, breathe. When swimming with fins, your arms play an important role in getting your head above the surface to breathe, but can also be valuable in adding some power to your stroke.

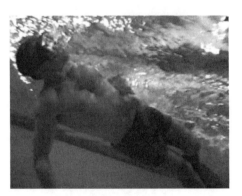

4. **Recovery.** As your bottom arm completes its stroke and is moving forward above your head, your top arm should be moving over your head just ahead of your bottom arm. Keep your top arm close to your body in order to reduce drag.

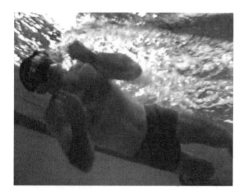 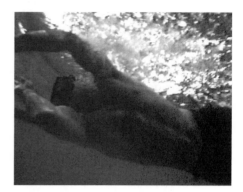

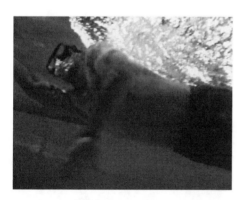 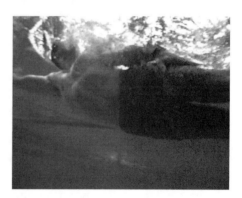

5. **Stretch before you swim.** It is extremely important to stretch your calves, ankles, and feet muscles/tendons before putting on your fins. You will lessen the amount of pain and fatigue in your feet and ankles if you stretch about 10-15 minutes before swimming over a mile in fins.

CRAWLSTROKE (FREESTYLE)

Hypoxic swim training. You will not use the crawlstroke much at BUD/S, but it is a great way to exercise and build your cardiovascular system, especially with hypoxic swimming workouts. The word hypoxic means low oxygen. Adapting this type of workout to swimming is easy, yet will probably be the most challenging cardiovascular exercise you will ever do. Hypoxic swimming easily compares to high-altitude training. Basically, your body is performing with less oxygen because of controlled breath holds while you surface swim. Instead of breathing every stroke or every other stroke, you will hold your breath for up to 10-12 strokes at a time. You will experience increased lactic acid levels, muscle fatigue, and an extremely high heart rate from hypoxic swimming, just as you would if you were running in the mountains. This gets your body used to performing with less oxygen, resulting in increased endurance when you swim regularly and breathe every stroke.

WARNING: Potentially dangerous—Do not perform alone!

Here are a few freestyle tips to help you increase your endurance and break up the monotony of sidestroke swimming.

1. **Kicking off the wall.** In pool swimming, kicking off the wall is essential to building up momentum and reducing the number of strokes per length. With your legs in a full squatting position against the wall, explode in the direction you are swimming and begin 6-inch flutter kicks. Keep your arms extended over your head. As your momentum decreases, begin the 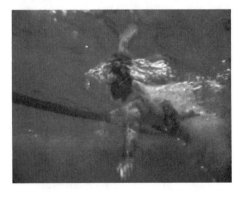 single arm pull, and surface to breathe. By this time you should be about 8-10 yards away from the wall.

2. **6-Inch Flutter kicks.** Using 6-inch flutter kicks will help you maintain a streamlined position in the water by keeping your body position horizontal. Constant flutter kicks are not necessary, but are recommended for short distance and endurance swimming like you will be doing in this workout.

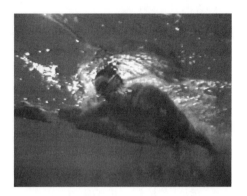

3. **Arm pulls.** An efficient arm pull is the most powerful and important part of swimming freestyle. The stroke begins with one arm extended over your head and ends when that arm is next to your hip. Each arm opposes the other and is never in the same position or moving in the same direction. As one arm is pulling through the stroke, the other is recovering forward.

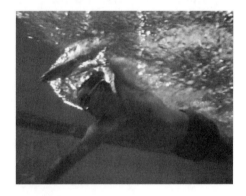

The arm pull is broken down into two parts: the pull and the push. As you pull one arm over your head, bend your elbow slightly and pull your arm under your body about 4-6 inches away from your chest. Once your hand is just below chest level, your pull stroke changes into a push stroke using the triceps muscles in your arm. From your chest, simply straighten out your arm until it brushes past your hips.

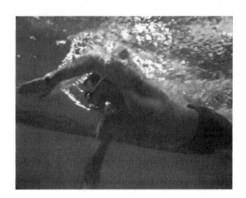

4. **Recovery:** Torso twist and high elbow. After a full arm stroke, recover the arm in front of you by getting your elbow high out of the water. This is aided by slightly twisting your torso in order to get your shoulder and arm out of the water. Breathing requires you to twist your torso at the end of your stroke. Your hand should be by your hip with your other hand extended over your head. This enables you to slightly turn your neck to breathe while still, and most importantly keeping your head in the water. Half of your face should still be underwater when you breathe. This is the most difficult part of freestyle to master—breathing and not lifting your head out of the water.

5. **Keep your head down.** Your body will act like a see-saw in the water. If your head comes out of the water, your lower body will sink, creating more drag and making your stroke much less efficient. A good rule of thumb is to make the water hit the hair line on your head as you glide through the water.

*The photos for this section were excerpted from the video Five Star Fitness Adventure: Navy SEAL Fitness: Preparing for the Teams. Techniques for mastering the sidestroke (with and without fins) and freestyle are detailed in full on this video, available from Five Star Fitness. For more information, please call 1-800-906-1234 or see the back pages of this book.

ROPE CLIMBING: JUST FOR FUN

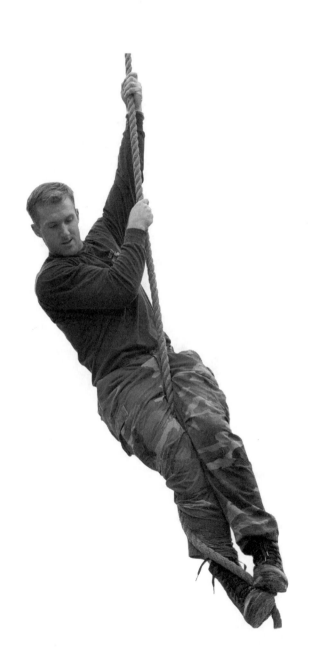

BASIC ROPE CLIMBING TECHNIQUES

Using your feet

Wrap the rope around your leg as follows: The top goes at the inner thigh, between your legs, around your knee and calf on the outside of your leg, and across the top of your boot. With the unwrapped leg, clamp your foot on to the rope on the opposite foot. This will act as a brake and you can actually support yourself without using your hands and arms.

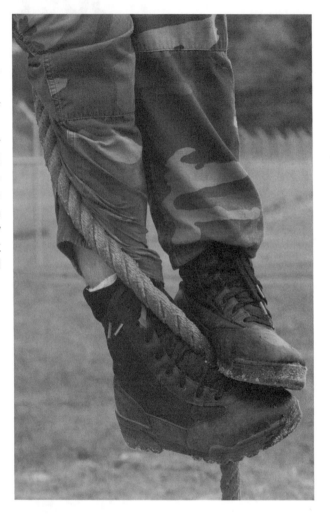

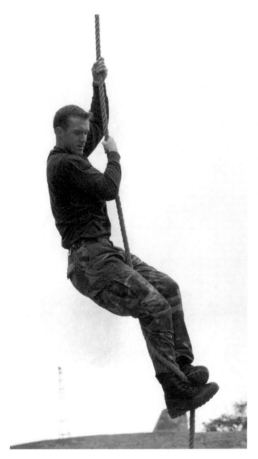

The technique to use so that you do not completely burn out your arms and grip is called the **Brake and Squat Technique.** Climb up the rope by bending your legs, sliding the rope across your foot by loosening the brake foot. Once you have moved about 1-1.5 feet of rope across your foot, brake and straighten your legs. Now you are using your legs to get you up the rope. This does require some amount of upper body strength but will save your energy for the most important part of rope climbing—GETTING DOWN!

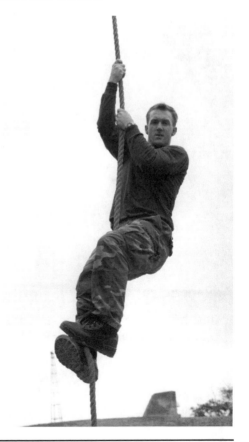

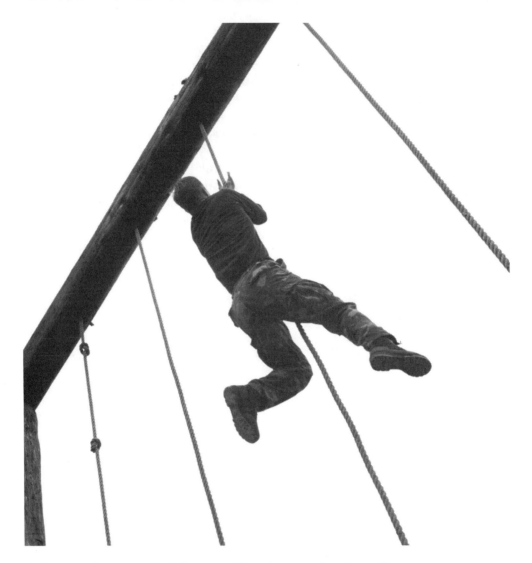

Advanced rope climbing—without your feet on the rope

This method of climbing a rope is a great workout and is absolutely exhausting. Your forearm muscles, biceps and back muscles will scream after a few times of climbing 30 feet of rope without using your legs.

Using a hand over hand method, slowly pull yourself up the rope about 6-12 inches at a time. This method requires an excellent grip (which you can first build by doing pull-ups) and biceps with stamina.

THE **12 WEEKS** TO **BUD/S** WORKOUT

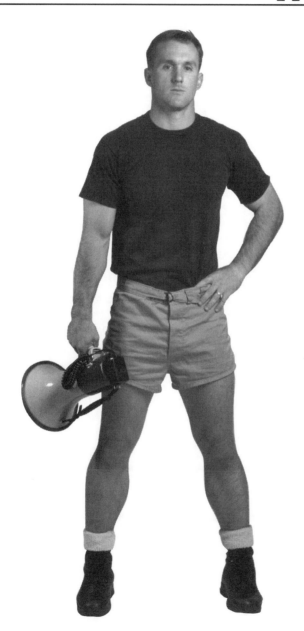

During the 12-week program, you will encounter many types of workouts. Each workout is designed to make you stronger in a different way. In the following pages, I've briefly explained each workout so you will have a better idea of what to expect during your 12 weeks of intense exercising. In the course of the 12-week program, the structure of the workouts will stay the same, but the difficulty of each workout will grow as the number of repetitions increases.

THE PT PYRAMID

This workout is deceivingly difficult. The PT Pyramid is unique from any other workout because it has a warm-up, maximum, and a cool down period built into it. Begin climbing the Pyramid on the left side of the base. The levels of the Pyramid are the number of repetitions required in each set. Some exercises will have a (x2) or a (x3) next to the name of the exercise. The repetition number on the pyramid is multiplied by this number, making the workout much more challenging. Usually three or four different exercises are involved in this type of workout.

For example, the first sets of this workout go in this order:

SET #1
> Pull-ups (x1) = 1 rep
> Pushups (x2) = 2 reps
> Crunches (x3) = 3 reps

SET #2
> Pull-ups (x1) = 2 reps
> Pushups (x2) = 4 reps
> Crunches (x3) = 6 reps
>> *And onto . . .*

SET #10
> Pull-ups (x1) = 10 reps
> Pushups (x2) = 20 reps
> Crunches (x3) = 30 reps

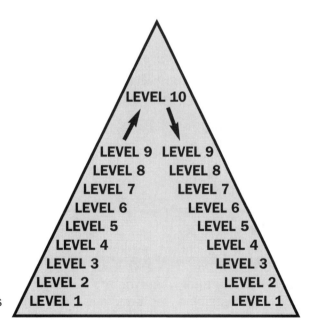

The 12 Weeks To BUD/S Workout

Once you reach the top of the pyramid, repeat the numbers and work your way down the right side until you are at the base of the pyramid again. Once you reach the bottom right side of the pyramid, you are finished. If you are beginning a workout program for the first time, do not go on to the following week's workouts until you can successfully complete the entire 19 sets of the pyramid workout.

THREE-MILE TRACK WORKOUT

The track workout is a great way to build speed and endurance for the 1.5-mile run as well as the 4-mile-timed run you will experience weekly at BUD/S. You will begin this interval training program by warming up with a steady one-mile run. This mile should be at a comfortable pace, usually a 7- to 8-minute mile. Run the next 1/4 mile at a full sprint; then jog another 1/4 mile at the same pace you ran the first mile. Repeat the 1/4-mile sprint and 1/4-jog again. Now repeat the same sprint/jog sequence with 1/8 miles four times, totaling another mile of interval training.

3-MILE TRACK WORKOUT		
1 mile jog (7:00-8:00 minute pace)	*then . . .*	1/4 mile sprint
1/4 mile jog (7:00-8:00 minute pace)	*then . . .*	1/4 mile sprint
1/4 mile jog (7:00-8:00 minute pace)	*then . . .*	1/8 mile sprint
1/8 mile jog	*then . . .*	1/8 mile sprint
1/8 mile jog	*then . . .*	1/8 mile sprint
1/8 mile jog	*then . . .*	1/8 mile sprint
1/8 mile jog		

This is not a walking workout. The object of interval training is to catch your breath from running while still moving at a jogging pace. This will speed your recovery time when you are resting. Quicker recovery time means you have more stamina and endurance, and will feel better after rigorous exercise than ever before.

If you have to build yourself up to the above workout by either decreasing the distance or speed, or walking during the jogging portion of the workout, that is fine! The object of this workout is to push yourself, but you can build a foundation by working your way up to the specified times and distances of the 3-Mile Track Workout.

HYPOXIC SWIM PYRAMID

•*Do not perform this workout alone.*•

The term hypoxic means low oxygen. By holding your breath and surface swimming (freestyle), you will receive a cardiovascular workout like no other. The only comparisons to hypoxic swimming are high-altitude running and cross-country skiing. The reason these workouts are similar is because exercise in high-altitudes, where there is less oxygen in the air, deprives your muscles of the oxygen you need. The same is true for holding your breath while swimming. Lactic acid and fatigue quickly build in your body as you exercise in low oxygen environments; therefore, you can get into much better shape in a shorter amount of time.

After training with a regimented hypoxic swim workout, when you swim normally (breathing every other stroke) your body will have become accustomed to not receiving sufficient oxygen. Thus, you will have more than enough oxygen to feed your muscles, and your performance will be greatly enhanced.

RUN / SWIM / RUN

The Run / Swim / Run workout is one of the best ways to build the endurance you will need for SEAL training. This lower body, cardiovascular exercise program will enable you to build the stamina and endurance needed for increasing your Navy SEAL PFT scores. The object of this workout is to run the specified distance as fast as you can and quickly start swimming with little transition time. After swimming, immediately begin running again, and try to match your pace from the first run of the workout.

SWIM-PT

The Swim-PT workout is a quick way to receive a great cardiovascular workout and build muscle stamina at the same time. The challenge of the

Swim-PT workout is to swim 100 meters, jump out of the pool, and immediately begin performing pushups and abdominal exercises. After the pushups and situps are completed, jump back in the water and swim 100 meters. Repeat the above sequence for the specified number of sets.

PULL-UP WORKOUT

Here's how it works:

	Regular	Reverse	Close	Wide	Mountain Climber Grip
Set #	1-5	6-10	11-15	16-20	21-25
Reps	2,4,6,8,10	2,4,6,8,10	2,4,6,8,10	2,4,6,8,10	2,4,6,8,10
Total	30 reps +	30 reps +	30 reps +	30 reps +	30 reps = 150 reps

The above workout is the most advanced pull-up workout of **The Complete Guide to Navy SEAL Fitness**, totaling 25 sets and 150 repetitions of pull-ups. Before you proceed to the next type of pull-ups, complete the 5 sets of 2, 4, 6, 8, 10 repetitions of the same type.

SUPER SETS

Most people have never done over 500 pushups and 500 situps in a 30-40 minute workout. Each set of six exercises should be completed within a two-minute period; therefore, the 20 super set workout should be finished within 40 minutes. For example, the 20 super set workout in week #3 is done the following way:

> **Set #1:** 10 Situps → 10 Pushups → 10 Atomic Situps → 10 Triceps Pushups → 10 Leg Levers → 10 Dive Bomber or Wide Grip Pushups
>
> Repeat sequence 19 times.

The total number of pushups and abdominal exercises in this workout is 600 (each!). This workout is sometimes referred to as the "Time-Saver" workout. If you are running short on time, you can finish 300 pushups and situps in just 20 minutes. If you are a beginner, I recommend you cut the number of supersets in half. You will still get 300 repetitions in your workout, but it is important to build a solid base for several months before you attempt to challenge yourself with 600 repetitions of any exercise.

LOWER BODY PT

If you are not used to exercising your legs, you must stretch before, during, and after Lower Body PT. These exercises are explosive and plyometric exercises designed to build speed, strength and endurance. In this workout, you will concentrate on exercises such as frog hops, jumpovers, and lunges, designed to build power in your legs. Whether you are running in boots on soft sand or swimming with fins in the ocean, you will need to have fit and strong legs. If you are not interested in SEAL training, Lower Body PT will build definition in your legs. Perform each exercise the specified number of repetitions, take 15 seconds to stretch, and repeat until all the exercises are complete.

PUSHUP / SITUP / DIP PYRAMID

The object of the Pushup / Situp / Dip Pyramid is to rapidly increase the repetitions in your workout. You will need to perform high repetitions at BUD/S and this is a great way to prepare for hundreds of pushups and situps. The workout goes like this: Begin with pushups and do 20 repetitions the first set. Then, alternate exercises and do 40 repetitions of situps. Next, quickly change to the dip position and perform 15 repetitions. Basically, you are climbing three pyramids at the same time, alternating exercises until you have reached the bottom right of all three pyramids. The toughest set is 50 pushups, 100 situps, and 30 dips.

MINIMAL RUNNING WEEK

Statistically, lower extremity injuries occur during the third week of any running program. Overuse (too much running) or improper preparation will definitely result in injuries to your shins, feet, knees, and/or hips. You should take advantage of this week and stretch well, rest, and ice your joints and shins. You will not get out of shape because you are not running. This week will be challenging because of the amount of swimming you will do to replace the cardiovascular running workout. If you are 100% healthy and an advanced athlete, you may ride a bike for up to one hour in addition to the swimming. It is recommended that you give your legs a break this week, because you will not get a rest in the upcoming weeks.

FREQUENTLY ASKED QUESTIONS

How long should I rest in between exercise sets or running and swimming sprints?

Rest as long as you need. Eventually, your rest times should decrease in time and frequency. A good goal is to try to rest about 15-20 seconds between pull-up sets. For the swimming sprints and hypoxic workout, try to rest a maximum of 30 seconds before starting again. For running sprints, the rest period will increase as your distance increases if you walk back to the starting line. A 100-yard sprint will give you more rest than a 20-yard sprint.

What strokes should I use during run/swim/run?

I recommend swimming as fast as you can. So try swimming freestyle. If you are training for BUD/S, use the sidestroke (with or without fins).

What counts as a stroke in the hypoxic swim workout?

A stroke in the hypoxic swim workout is one arm movement. When you pull with both arms doing freestyle, that counts as two strokes. The hardest part of this workout is not breathing during the increasing number of strokes.

I'm having trouble in week four. Should I skip to week five?

Yes, if you feel like it. If you are having problems with just one exercise, go on to the next week. If you are having problems with running, swimming, and pull-ups, you may want to repeat the week causing trouble.

Now you are ready to begin.

Turn the page to face Week #1,
and the 12-week challenge...

Week #1

MONDAY

SEAL PFT

500-yd swim: sidestroke
  or breaststroke
pushups: max in 2 min.
situps: max in 2 min.
Pull-ups: max (no time
  limit)
1.5-mile run: Run in
  combat boots and pants

TUESDAY

Swimming

200m warmup
500m sidestroke
3 x 100m sprints with 20
sec. rest
200m cool down

WEDNESDAY

Running

3-mile timed run
  (sprint 1.5 miles, jog 1.5
  miles)

THURSDAY

Swimming

200m warmup
1000m sidestroke
200m cool down

Upper Body PT

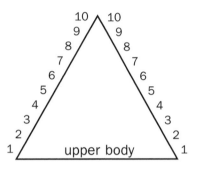

Pull-ups x 1
Pushups x 2
Situps x 3
each level of the pyramid

Neck exercises

up/down: 20
left/right: 20

8-count Body Builders: 10

Max pushups in 2 min.
Max situps in 2 min.
Max pull-ups

FRIDAY

Running

4-mile timed run

SATURDAY

Swimming

200m warmup
1000m sidestroke
200m cool down

Week #2

MONDAY

Upper Body PT

Pull-ups   (sets x reps)
  Regular grip   2 x 7
  Reverse grip   2 x 7
  Close grip   2 x 7
  Wide grip   2 x 7
  Mountain climbers 2 x 7
Pushups   (sets x reps)
  Regular   2 x 15
  Triceps   2 x 10
  Wide   2 x 15
  Dive Bomber   2 x 15
Dips   2 x 15
Arm Haulers   3 x 30

Neck exercises

  up/down: 25
  left/right: 25

Abdominal PT

Do two cycles of:
  Regular situps   40
  4-way crunches   40
  (Regular, Reverse,
  Left, and Right: 40 of
  each)
  Leg levers   40
  Flutter kicks   50
  1/2 situps   40
  Stretch 1 min.

Running

3-mile timed run (sprint
  1.5 miles, jog 1.5
  miles)

TUESDAY

Swimming

200m warmup
500m sidestroke
3 x 100m sprints
4 x 50m sprints
200m cool down

WEDNESDAY

Upper Body PT

Pull-ups   (sets x reps)
  Regular grip   2 x 7
  Reverse grip   2 x 7
  Close grip   2 x 7
  Wide grip   2 x 7
  Mountain climbers 2 x 7
Pushups   (sets x reps)
  Regular   2 x 15
  Triceps   2 x 10
  Wide   2 x 15
  Dive Bomber   2 x 15
Dips   2 x 15
Arm Haulers   3 x 30
8-count Body Builders   15

Neck exercises

  up/down: 25
  left/right: 25

Abdominal PT

Do two cycles of:
  Regular situps   40
  4-way crunches   40
  (Regular, Reverse,
  Left, and Right:
  40 of each)
  Leg levers   40
  Flutter kicks   50
  1/2 situps   40
  Stretch 1 min.

Running

4-mile timed run

THURSDAY

Swimming

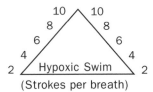

(Strokes per breath)

10 x 50m freestyle with 10 sec. interval (rest) in between each 50m (Each level of the pyramid is 50m).

DO NOT SWIM ALONE!

Running

3-mile Track Workout
Jog: 1 mile in 7 min.
Sprint: 1/4 mile
Jog: 1/4 mile in 2 min.
Sprint: 1/4 mile
Jog: 1/4 mile in 2 min.
Sprint: 1/8 mile
Jog: 1/8 mile in 1 min.
Sprint: 1/8 mile
Jog: 1/8 mile in 1 min.
Sprint: 1/8 mile
Jog: 1/8 mile in 1 min.
Sprint: 1/8 mile
Jog: 1/8 mile in 1 min.

FRIDAY

Lower Body PT

Squats	3 x 10
Lunges	3 x 10
Frog Hops	3 x 10
Heel Raises	3 x 15
Jumpovers	3 x 15

Sprints

20m 1/2 pace x 2
20m full sprint x 2
40m 3/4 pace x 2
60m full sprint x 4
100m 1/2 pace x 1
100m full sprint x 2

Neck exercises

up/down: 25
left/right: 25

SATURDAY

Swimming

200m warmup
500m sidestroke
3 x 100m sprints (side)
4 x 50m sprints (side)
200m cool down

Running

3-mile timed run

Pull-ups 5 x 2,4,6,8 reps

Regular grip
Reverse grip
Close grip
Wide grip
Mountain climbers
Total Pull-ups = 100

Abdominal PT

Do two cycles of:

Regular situps	40
4-way crunches (40 each way)	40
Leg levers	40
Flutter kicks	50
1/2 situps	40
Stretch 1 min.	

8-count Body Builders 15

Max pushups in 2 min.
Max situps in 2 min.
Max pull-ups

MONDAY

Swim/PT

10 sets of:
  100m freestyle
  20 pushups
  20 abs of choice

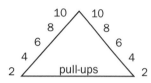

Dips: 25, 20, 15, 10

Neck exercises

up/down: 25
left/right: 25

No running: Due to common overuse injuries such as shin splints and stress fractures, take this week off even if you feel fine.

TUESDAY

Swimming

200m warmup
500m with fins
500m without fins
3 x 100m freestyle sprints
  at 1 min. 45 sec.
200m cool down

WEDNESDAY

Swim/PT

10 sets of:
  100m freestyle
  20 pushups
  20 abs of choice

Pull-ups 5 x 2,4,6,8 reps

Regular grip
Reverse grip
Close grip
Wide grip
Mountain climbers

Neck exercises

up/down: 25
left/right: 25

THURSDAY

Swimming

200m warmup
500m with fins
500m without fins
3 x 100m freestyle sprints
    at 1 min. 45 sec.
200m cool down

FRIDAY

Swim/PT

10 sets of:
    100m freestyle
    20 pushups
    20 abs of choice

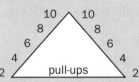

10   10
  8   8
  6   6
  4   4
2   pull-ups   2

Dips: 25,20,15,10

Neck exercises

up/down: 25
left/right: 25

SATURDAY

Running

3-mile timed run
(sprint 1.5 miles,
    jog 1.5 miles)

Swimming

200m warmup
500m with fins
500m without fins

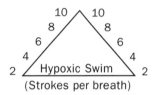

10   10
  8   8
  6   6
  4   4
2   Hypoxic Swim   2
(Strokes per breath)

10 x 50m freestyle sprints
    at 1 min. 45 sec.
200m cool down

DO NOT SWIM ALONE!

Lower Body PT

Exercise	Sets/Reps
Squats	3 x 15
Lunges	3 x 15
Heel Raises	3 x 15
Dirty Dogs	50

Week #4

SEAL PFT

500yd swim: sidestroke
   or breaststroke
pushups: max in 2 min.
situps: max in 2 min.
pull-ups: max (no time
   limit)
1.5 mile run: Run in
   combat boots and pants

Run-Swim-Run

Run: 3 miles < 21 min.
Swim: 1 mile with fins
   < 30 min.
Run: 3 miles < 21 min.
Total Time = 1 hr. 15 min.

Neck exercises

up/down: 35
left/right: 35

Upper Body PT

Pull-ups 5 x 2,4,6,8 reps
   Regular grip
   Reverse grip
   Close grip
   Wide grip
   Mountain climbers
Total Pull-ups = 100

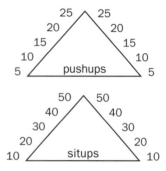

8 count Body Builders: 20

Max pushups in 2 min.
Max situps in 2 min.
Max pull-ups

THURSDAY

Lower Body PT

Squats	10,15,20
Lunges	10,15,20
Frog Hops	10,15,20
Heel Raises	10,15,20
(each leg)	
Jumpovers	10,15,20
Dirty Dogs	100
(each leg)	

Neck exercises

up/down: 35
left/right: 35

Springs

20m 1/2 pace x 2
20m full sprint x 3
40m 3/4 pace x 2
40m full sprint x 3
60m full sprint x 5
80m full sprint x 4
100m full sprint x 3

Swimming

200m warmup
500m sidestroke
500m freestyle
500m with fins
200m cool down

FRIDAY

Running

5 miles < 35 min.

SATURDAY

Upper Body PT

Pull-ups 5 x 2,4,6,8 reps
  Regular grip
  Reverse grip
  Close grip
  Wide grip
  Mountain climbers
Total Pull-ups = 100

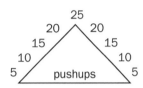

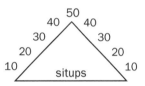

Neck exercises

up/down: 35
left/right: 35

8-count Body Builders: 20
Max pushups in 2 min.
Max situps in 2 min.
Max pull-ups

Swimming

2000m with fins

Week #5

MONDAY	TUESDAY	WEDNESDAY

MONDAY

20 Super Sets:

Triceps Pushups	10
Regular Situps	7
Pushups	10
Reverse Crunches	7
Wide Pushups	10
1/2 Situps	7

Do 20 cycles of all six exercises. You have 2 min. to perform each cycle.
Total time: 40 min.
Total Pushups: 600
Total Abs: 420

Upper Body PT

Pull-ups: 16, 14, 12
Dips: 25, 20, 15
8-count Body Builders: 20, 15, 10

Neck Exercises:

up/down: 40
left/right: 40

Swimming

Swim with fins: 30 min.
Swim continuously for at least 1 mile

TUESDAY

Run-Swim-Run

3-mile run
1-mile swim without fins
3-mile run

WEDNESDAY

Lower Body PT

Squats	3 x 15
Lunges	3 x 15
Frog Hops	2 x 10
Jumpovers	2 x 20
Heel Raises	3 x 20
Dirty Dogs	3 x 50

Sprints

20m x 5
40m x 5
60m x 5
100m x 4
200m x 2
440m x 1

Swimming

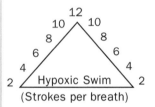
(Strokes per breath)

11 x 100m freestyle without fins. 15 sec. rest in between each 100m.
DO NOT SWIM ALONE!

Neck exercises:

up/down: 40
left/right: 40

THURSDAY

Upper Body PT

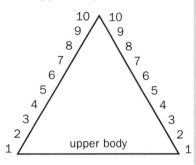

Pull-ups x 1
Pushups x 2
Abs of choice x 3
Dips x 2
Each level of the pyramid

Flutter kicks 100
Leg Levers 100
8-count Body Builders 25

Neck exercises:

up/down: 40
left/right: 40

Run-Swim-Run

3-mile run
1-mile swim without fins
3-mile run

FRIDAY

Swimming

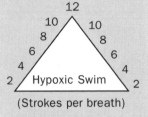

(Strokes per breath)

11 x 100 freestyle without fins. 15 sec. rest in between each 100m.

DO NOT SWIM ALONE!

Running

3-mile Track Workout
Jog 1 mile in 7 min.
Sprint 1/4 mile
Jog 1/4 mile in 2 min.
Sprint 1/4 mile
Jog 1/4 mile in 2 min.
Sprint 1/8 mile
Jog 1/8 mile in 1 min.
Sprint 1/8 mile
Jog 1/8 mile in 1 min.
Sprint 1/8 mile
Jog 1/8 mile in 1 min.
Sprint 1/8 mile
Jog 1/8 mile in 1 min.

SATURDAY

Upper Body PT

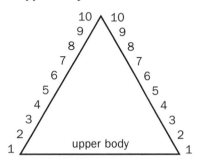

Pull-ups x 1
Pushups x 2
Abs of choice x 3
Dips x 2
Each level of the pyramid

Flutter kicks 100
Leg Levers 100

Neck exercises:

up/down: 40
left/right: 40

Week #6

MONDAY

10 Super Sets

Pull-ups	8
Pushups	20
Abs of choice	20
Dips	10

Abs Super Set x 2

Hanging Knee Ups	10
Regular situps	30
Oblique crunch (left and right) 30 each side	30
Atomic situps	30
Crunches	30
Reverse crunches	30

Neck exercises:

up/down: 40
left/right: 40

Swimming

Swim continuously for 45
min. with fins.
Goal: 1.5-2 miles

Running

4-mile Track Workout
Jog 1 mile in 7 mins.
3 sets of:
  Sprint 1/4 mile
  Jog 1/4 mile in 1 min.
  45 sec.
6 sets of:
  Sprint 1/8 mile
  Jog 1/8 mile in 1 min.

TUESDAY

Swimming

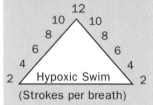

Hypoxic Swim
(Strokes per breath)

11 x 150m freestyle
without fins. 15
sec. rest in
between each 200m

DO NOT SWIM ALONE!

WEDNESDAY

Lower Body PT

Squats	4 x 15
Lunges	4 x 15
Frog Hops	3 x 15
Jumpovers	3 x 20
Heel Raises	4 x 20
Dirty Dogs	2 x 100

Sprints

20m x 5
40m x 5
60m x 5
100m x 5
200m x 3
440m x 2

Swimming

Swim continuously for 45
min. with fins
Goal: 1.5-2 miles

Running

4-mile Track Workout
Jog 1 mile in 7 min.
3 sets of:
  Sprint 1/4 mile
  Jog 1/4 mile in 1 min.
  45 sec.
6 sets of:
  Sprint 1/8 mile
  Jog 1/8 mile in 1 min.

THURSDAY

10 Super Sets

Pull-ups	8
Pushups	20
Abs of choice	20
Dips	10

8-count Body Builders: 5
Max pushups in 2 min.
Max situps in 2 min.
Max pull-ups

Neck exercises:

up/down: 40
left/right: 40

Abs Super Set x 2

Hanging Knee Ups	10
Regular situps	30
Oblique crunch	30
(left and right)	
30 each side	
Atomic situps	30
Crunches	30
Reverse crunches	30

Swimming

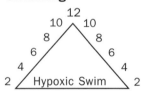

11 x 150m freestyle without fins. 15 sec. rest in between each 200m.

FRIDAY

Swimming

Swim continuously for 45 min. with fins.
Goal: 1.5-2 miles

SATURDAY

Upper Body PT

Pull-ups: 4 x 2, 4, 6, 8, 10
Regular grip
Reverse grip
Close grip
Wide grip

Pushups: 50,40,30,20,10
Dips: 30,25,20,15,10
8-count Body Builders:
25,20,15,10

Max pushups in 2 min.
Max situps in 2 min.
Max pull-ups

Neck exercises:

up/down: 40
left/right: 40

Abs Super Set x 2

Flutter kicks 100
Leg Levers 100
Situps 100

Week #7

MONDAY

SEAL PFT

500yd swim: sidestroke or
   breaststroke
pushups: max in 2 min.
situps: max in 2 min.
pull-ups: max (no time
   limit)
1.5 mile run: Run in
   combat boots and pants

TUESDAY

Run-Swim-Run

Run 4 miles
Swim 3000m with fins
Run 3 miles

Lower Body PT

Squats	3 x 15
Lunges	3 x 15
Frog Hops	2 x 10
Jumpovers	2 x 20
Heel Raises	3 x 20
Dirty Dogs	3 x 50

Neck exercises:

   up/down: 50
   left/right: 50

WEDNESDAY

Swimming

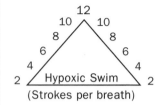

11 x 200m freestyle
   without fins. 15 sec.
   rest in between each
   200m.

DO NOT SWIM ALONE!

THURSDAY

Upper Body PT

Pull-ups:

Regular grip	2 x 7
Reverse grip	2 x 7
Close grip	2 x 7
Wide grip	2 x 7
Mountain climbers	2 x 7

Pushups:

Regular	2 x 30
Triceps	2 x 20
Wide	2 x 30
Dive Bomber	2 x 30

Dips	2 x 25
Arm Haulers	3 x 50
8-count	
Body Builders	2 x 20

Max pushups in 2 min.
Max situps in 2 min.
Max pull-ups

Neck exercises

up/down: 50
left/right: 50

Abs Super Set x 2:

Regular situps	60
4-way crunches	50
Leg levers	60
Flutter kicks	150
1/2 situps	100
Stretch 1 min.	

Running

5-mile timed run

Swimming

1 mile swim with fins

FRIDAY

Running

Run 6 miles.

SATURDAY

Run-Swim/PT-Run

Run 4 miles.
15 sets: Swim/PT
   20 pushups
   20 abs of choice
   100m swim
Run 3 miles.

MONDAY

Upper Body PT

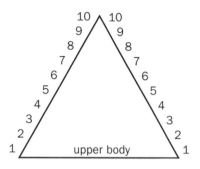

Pull-ups x 1
Pushups x 3
Abs of choice x 5
Dips x 2

Run-Swim-Run

Run 4 miles.
Swim 1 mile with fins.
Run 3 miles.

Neck exercises:

up/down: 2 x 35
left/right: 2 x 35

TUESDAY

Lower Body PT

Squats	4 x 20
Lunges	4 x 20
Frog Hops	3 x 20
Jumpovers	3 x 20
Heel Raises	4 x 20
Dirty Dogs	2 x 100

Running

4-mile Track Workout
Jog 1 mile in 7 min.
3 sets of:
   Sprint 1/4 mile in
      1 min. 20 sec.
   Jog 1/4 mile in
      1 min. 45 sec.
6 sets of:
   Sprint 1/8 mile in 40
   sec.
   Jog 1/8 mile in 1 min.

Swimming

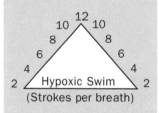

11 x 200m freestyle
   without fins. 15 sec.
   rest in between each
   200m.

DO NOT SWIM ALONE!

WEDNESDAY

Swimming

Swim with fins 1.5 miles.

Neck exercises

up/down: 2 x 35
left/right: 2 x 35

THURSDAY

Run-Swim/PT-Run

Run 3 miles.
10 sets: Swim/PT
   100m sprints
   25 pushups
   25 abs of choice
Run 3 miles.

Max pushups in 2 min.
Max situps in 2 min.
Max pull-ups

FRIDAY

Upper Body PT

Pull-ups: 5 x 2,4,6,8,10
   Regular grip
   Reverse grip
   Close grip
   Wide grip
   Mountain climber
Total Pull-ups: 150

Arm Haulers: 2 x 75

Neck exercises:

   up/down: 2 x 35
   left/right: 2 x 35

Abs Super Set

Flutter kicks 150
Leg Levers 150
Situps 150

Swimming

Swim with fins 1.5 miles.

Running

Run 4 miles in 27 min.,
   in sand if available.

SATURDAY

Running

Run 6 miles within 40 min.

Upper Body PT

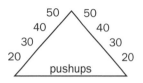

pushups

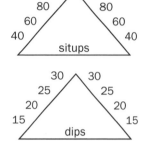

situps

dips

Week #9

Upper Body PT

Pull-ups: 5 x 2,4,6,8,10
- Regular grip
- Reverse grip
- Close grip
- Wide grip
- Mountain climber

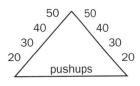

pushups

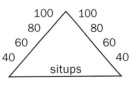

situps

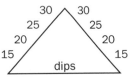

dips

Arm Haulers: 2 x 75

Neck exercises:

up/down: 2 x 40
left/right: 2 x 40

Run-Swim-Run

Run 4 miles.
Swim 1 mile with fins.
Run 3 miles.

Lower Body PT

Squats	4 x 20
Lunges	4 x 20
Frog Hops	3 x 20
Jumpovers	3 x 20
Heel Raises	4 x 20
Dirty Dogs	2 x 100

Sprints

20m x 5
40m x 5
60m x 5
100m x 5
200m x 3
440m x 2

Swimming

200m warmup
500m pulls (no kick)
300m kicks (no pull)
8 x 50m sprints
   (15 sec. rest
   between each)
2 x 100m sprints
   (20 sec. rest
   between each)
Hypoxic: 4,6,8,10
   (strokes/breath)
   x 100m
200m cool down

Run-Swim-Run

Run 4 miles.
Swim 1 mile with fins.
Run 4 miles.

Neck exercises

up/down: 2 x 40
left/right: 2 x 40

THURSDAY

Swimming

200m warmup
500m pulls (no kick)
300m kicks (no pull)
8 x 50m sprints
  (15 sec. rest between
  each)
2 x 100m sprints
  (20 sec. rest between
  each)
Hypoxic: 4,6,8,10
 (strokes/breath) x 100m
200m cool down

FRIDAY

Lower Body PT

Squats	4 x 20
Lunges	4 x 20
Frog Hops	3 x 20
Jumpovers	3 x 20
Heel Raises	4 x 20
Dirty Dogs	2 x 100

Running

Run 4 miles in 27 min.

Swimming

Swim 2000m with fins.

SATURDAY

Upper Body PT

Pull-ups: 5 x 2,4,6,8,10
  Regular grip
  Reverse grip
  Close grip
  Wide grip
  Mountain climbers

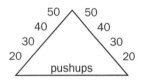

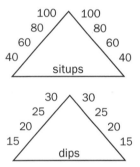

Neck exercises

up/down: 2 x 40
left/right: 2 x 40

Running

3-mile timed run.
(spring 1.5 mile, jog 1.5
  mile)

Week #10

MONDAY

SEAL PFT

500yd swim: sidestroke or
  breaststroke
pushups: max in 2 min.
situps: max in 2 min.
pull-ups: max (no time
  limit)
1.5 mile run: Run in
  combat boots and pants

TUESDAY

Running

Run 4 miles in 27 min.

WEDNESDAY

Upper Body PT

Pull-ups: 2,4,6,8,10 x 5
  Regular grip
  Reverse grip
  Close grip
  Wide grip

Arm Haulers: 2 x 75

20 Super Sets

Situps	10
Pushups	10
Atomic situps	10
Triceps	10
Leg Levers	10
Dive Bombers	10

Run-Swim-Run

Run 3 miles.
Swim 1 mile with fins.
Run 3 miles.

THURSDAY

Lower Body PT

Squats	3 x 20
Lunges	3 x 20
Frog Hops	3 x 15
Jumpovers	3 x 20
Heel Raises	3 x 20
Dirty Dogs	2 x 100

Sprints

20m x 5
40m x 5
60m x 5
100m x 5
200m x 3
440m x 2

FRIDAY

Running

Run 5 miles in 33 min.

SATURDAY

Swim/PT

15 sets of:
   Freestyle springs: 100m
   Pushups: 15
   Abs of choice: 15

Max pushups in 2 min.
Max situps in 2 min.
Max pull-ups

Arm Haulers: 2 x 75

Swimming

Swim 2 miles with fins.

Week #11

MONDAY

Upper Body PT

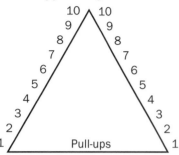

10 10
9 9
8 8
7 7
6 6
5 5
4 4
3 3
2 2
1 Pull-ups 1

25 Super Sets

Situps	10
Pushups	10
Atomic situps	10
Triceps	10
Leg Levers	10
Dive Bombers	10

Neck exercises:

up/down: 2 x 50
left/right: 2 x 50

Swimming

1-mile swim with fins

TUESDAY

Running

4-mile timed run

WEDNESDAY

Swim/PT

Hypoxic swim
5 x 50 at 50 sec. intervals
(6 strokes/breath)
4 x 50 at 55 sec. intervals
(8 strokes/breath)
3 x 50 at 1 min. intervals
(10 strokes/breath)
2 x 50 at 1 min. intervals
(12 strokes/breath)
1 x 50 (no breaths)

DO NOT DO ALONE!

Swim PT

10 Sets of:
100m sprint (freestyle)
15 pushups
15 abs of choice

Neck exercises:

up/down: 2 x 50
left/right: 2 x 50

THURSDAY

Running

4-mile timed run

FRIDAY

Swimming

1-mile swim with fins

Upper Body PT

Pull-ups: 5 x 2,4,6,8,10
  Regular grip
  Reverse grip
  Close grip
  Wide grip

Arm Haulers: 2 x 75

Neck exercises:

  up/down: 2 x 50
  left/right: 2 x 50

20 Super Sets

Situps	10
Pushups	10
Atomic situps	10
Triceps	10
Leg Levers	10
Dive Bombers	10

SATURDAY

Running

3-mile timed run
  (sprint 1.5 mile, jog 1.5 mile)

Week #12

MONDAY

20 Super Sets

Triceps Pushups	10
Regular Situps	7
Regular Pushups	10
Reverse Crunches	7
Wide Pushups	10
1/2 Situps	7

Total Time: 40 min.
Total Pushups: 600
Total Abs: 420

Pull-ups: 16, 14, 12
Dips: 25, 20, 15

Running

4-mile timed run

TUESDAY

Swimming

Hypoxic swim
5 x 50m,
  50 sec. intervals
4 x 50m,
  55 sec. intervals
3 x 50m,
  1 min. intervals
2 x 50m,
  1 min. intervals
1 x 50m

DO NOT SWIM ALONE!

The number of breaths per 50m = number of times you swim the 50m; i.e., 5 x 50m means you swim 50 meters five times on only 5 breaths...

WEDNESDAY

Running

4-mile timed run

THURSDAY

Swim/PT

10 sets of:
   100m freestyle sprint
   20 pushups
   20 abs of choice

Upper Body PT

Pull-ups: 5 x 2,4,6,8,10
   Regular grip
   Reverse grip
   Close grip
   Wide grip

Arm Haulers: 2 x 75

FRIDAY

Running

3-mile timed run

SATURDAY

Swimming

Hypoxic swim
   5 x 50m,
   50 sec. interval
   4 x 50m,
   55 sec. interval
   3 x 50m,
   1 min. interval
   2 x 50m,
   1 min. interval
   1 x 50m

DO NOT SWIM ALONE!

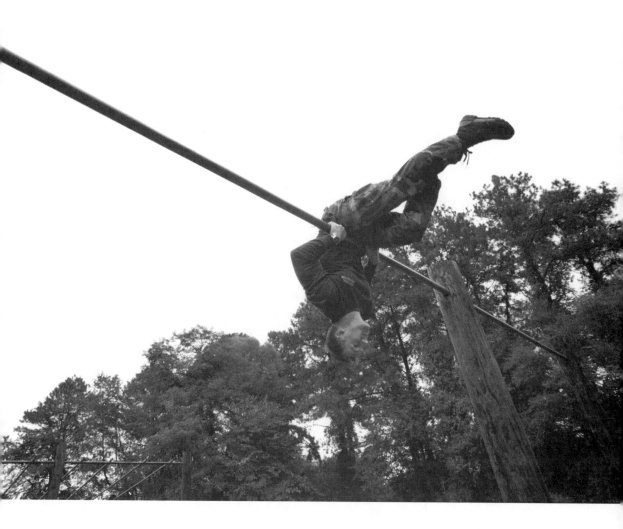

IF YOU ARE A BEGINNER...

If You Are A Beginner...

This workout is not specifically designed for people who are out of shape. However, you can alter some of the workouts to build a foundation in order to move on to the more challenging 12-week workout. First, you can test your level of fitness by taking the SEAL PFT.

500 yard swim—If you score above 13 minutes or do not complete:

1. Check your technique by reading Chapter 6 on swimming.
2. Build cardiovascular strength by running, biking, or hypoxic swimming (see Week #2 of the 12-week workout, Thursday).

1.5 mile run—If you score above 13 minutes or do not complete:

1. Check your technique by reading Chapter 5 on running.
2. Do the 3-mile Track Workout (see Week #2 of the 12-week workout, Thursday), except change the words "sprint/jog" to "run/walk."

Pull-ups—If you do less than 3 pull-ups:

1. Do negatives to build upper body strength. A negative is half of a complete repetition. Simply put your chin above the pull-up bar by stepping up to the bar. Then, slowly let yourself down to the starting position counting to 5. By fighting gravity on the downward motion of the pull-up, you are getting your muscles used to lifting your body weight. Eventually, you will be able to lift yourself over the bar.

Pushups—If you do less than 30 pushups in 2 minutes:

1. Do negatives until you can do a full pushup.
2. Do pushups on your knees.

Situps—If you do less than 30 situps in 2 minutes:

1. Do crunches, especially if you have lower back problems.

If you still cannot pass the minimum physical standards on the Navy SEAL

PFT, you will need to start with the four-week Pre-Training Workout. This is a four-week program that will help you build a foundation of strength and endurance. The workouts may be repetitious, but the best way to build the muscular stamina needed to pass the Navy SEAL PFT is by following these simple steps and finishing the four-week program.

Some general guidelines:

1. Work out five days a week and stretch two times every day.

2. Push yourself until you can no longer perform any of the exercises, and then resort to negative repetitions. Pushing yourself to total muscle failure will quickly increase your scores in pull-ups, pushups, and situps.

3. When running or swimming during the Pre-Training phase, concentrate more on perfecting your technique than on decreasing your times.

4. Stretch for 15 minutes after every workout in order to decrease your pain and soreness the following day.

Follow this workout program and you will be surprised that doing 300 pushups and over 500 crunches in one workout isn't as tough as you thought. After your four-week training program is complete, take the SEAL PFT again and strive to surpass the minimum scores (see page 21).

GOOD LUCK!

Week #1

Upper Body PT

Regular Pushups 2 x max
  (Do negatives if you
  have to, but stay off
  your knees!)
Wide Pushups 2 x max
Triceps Pushups 2 x max
Regular Pull-ups
  Do a pyramid to your
  max (for example, if
  your max is 5, do
  1,2,3,4,5)
Reverse Pull-ups
  Pyramid down to 1
  from your max
Regular Crunches 2 x 25
Reverse Crunches 2 x 25
Left and Right Crunches
  2 x 50 each side

Max pushups in 1 min.
Max situps in 1 min.
Max pull-ups (no time
  limit)

Lower Body PT

Squats	2 x 10
Lunges (each leg)	2 x 10
Heel Raises (each leg)	2 x 10
Frog Hops	1 x 5

Sprints

20 yd x 5
40 yd x 5
60 yd x 3

Jog 1 mile.
Stretch legs for 15 min.

Running

Jog 1/4 mile.
Stretch 10 min.
1.5-mile timed run.
Jog 1/4 mile.
Stretch 15 min.

THURSDAY

Swimming

Stretch 10 min.
500 yd. sidestroke or
  breaststroke, timed
500 yd sidestroke
  technique swim;
  concentrate on
  technique!
Read Chapter 6 on
  swimming.

FRIDAY

Run/Swim PT

Jog 1/4 mile
Stretch 10 min.
1.5-mile timed run

100 yd swim (freestyle)
10 pushups
10 situps
Repeat sequence 10
times!

SATURDAY

REST!

Week #2

Upper Body PT

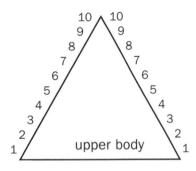

Pull-ups x 1
Pushups x 2
Situps x 3
Dips x 2
Each level of the pyramid

Running

Jog 1/4 mile
Stretch for 10 min.
2-mile timed run
Jog 1/4 mile
Stretch for 10 min.

Lower Body PT

Squats	2 x 15
Lunges (each leg)	2 x 15
Heel Raises (each leg)	2 x 15
Frog Hops	1 x 8

Sprints

20 yd x 5
40 yd x 4
60 yd x 3
100 yd x 2

Swimming

500 yds sidestroke
Stretch 10 min.

Running

Jog 1/4 mile
Stretch 10 min.
2-mile timed run
Jog 1/4 mile
Stretch 10 min.

THURSDAY

Same workout as Monday of this week, but swim 500 yds instead of running—give your legs a break!

After you swim:
  Max pushups in 1 min.
  Max situps in 1 min.
  Max pull-ups (no time limit)

FRIDAY

Running

Jog 1/4 mile
Stretch 10 min.
2-mile timed run
Jog 1/4 mile
Stretch 10 min.

SATURDAY

REST!

Week #3

MONDAY

Upper Body PT

Pull-ups:
1,2,3,4,5...max, and then back down to 1 (15 sec. break in between pull-ups)

10 Super Sets

Regular Pushups	5
Regular Crunches	10
Wide Pushups	5
Reverse Crunches	10
Triceps Pushups	5
1/2 Situps	10

Repeat this sequence 10 times, for a total of 150 pushups and 300 abdominal exercises. You have 2 min. to complete each set. If you finish in 1 min. 30 sec., you have 30 sec. rest before the next set.

Running

Jog 1/4 mile
Stretch 10 min.
2-mile timed run
Jog 1/4 mile
Stretch 10 min.

TUESDAY

Running

3-mile timed run

Swimming

800 yd swim

WEDNESDAY

Lower Body PT

Squats	3 x 15
Lunges	3 x 15
Heel Raises	3 x 15
Frog Hops	2 x 8

Sprints

20 yd x 5
40 yd x 4
60 yd x 3
100 yd x 2
220 yd x 1

THURSDAY

Upper Body PT

Pull-ups: 1,2,3,4,5...max;
  then back down to 1
  (15 sec. break in
  between pull-ups)

15 Super Sets

Regular Pushups	5
Regular Crunches	10
Wide Pushups	5
Reverse Crunches	10
Triceps Pushups	5
1/2 Situps	10

Repeat sequence 15
  times,
  for a total of 225
  pushups and 450
  abdominal exercises.

Swimming

500 yd swim

FRIDAY

Running

Jog 1/4 mile
Stretch 10 min.
3-mile timed run
Jog 1/4 mile
Stretch 10 min.

SATURDAY

REST!

Week #4

Upper Body PT

Pull-ups: 1,2,3,4,5 . . .
    max; then back down to
    1 (15 sec. break in
    between pull-ups)

15 Super Sets

Regular Pushups	5
Regular Crunches	10
Wide Pushups	5
Reverse Crunches	10
Triceps Pushups	5
1/2 Situps	10

Repeat sequence 15
    times,
    for a total of 225
    pushups and 450
    abdominal exercises.

Running

2-3 miles at a comfortable
    pace

Running

Jog 1/4 mile
Stretch 10 min.
3-mile timed run

Swimming

1000 yds sidestroke
Stretch 10 min.

Lower Body PT

Squats	3 x 15
Lunges	3 x 15
Heel Raises	3 x 15
Frog Hops	2 x 8

Sprints

20 yd x 5
40 yd x 4
60 yd x 3
100 yd x 2
220 yd x 1

THURSDAY

Upper Body PT

Pull-ups: 1,2,3,4,5 . . .
  max; then back down to
  1 (15 sec. break in
  between pull-ups)

20 Super Sets

Regular Pushups	5
Regular Crunches	10
Wide Pushups	5
Reverse Crunches	10
Triceps Pushups	5
1/2 Situps	10

Repeat sequence 200
  times,
  for a total of 300
  pushups and 600
  abdominal exercises.

Swimming

500 yds sidestroke

FRIDAY

Running

Jog 1/4 mile
Stretch 10 min.
4-mile timed run
Jog 1/4 mile
Stretch 10 min.

When you have completed the 4-week training program, take the SEAL PFT again. You will be surprised at how much your scores will improve. But don't stop there!

After you achieve the minimum scores, I encourage you to keep training, using the 12-week workout. You will soon be in the best physical shape of your life!

STEW'S TOP TEN LIST

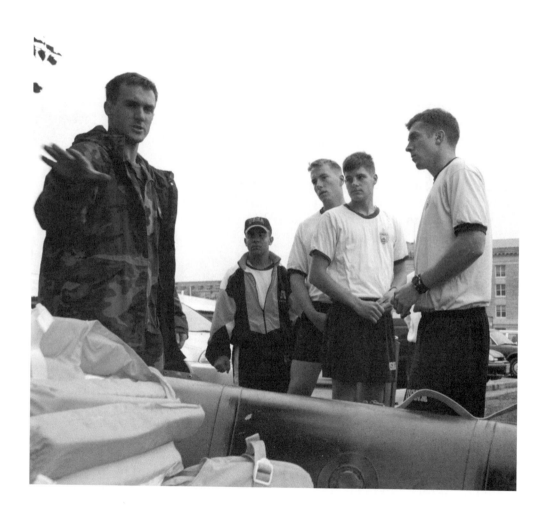

The Top Ten Before BUD/S

HERE ARE THE TOP TEN THINGS YOU NEED TO DO BEFORE YOU GO TO BUD/S

1. **Arrive fit!** Not just able to do the minimum scores but Stew Smith's recommend PFT scores:

500 yds swim	under 9:00
Pushups	100 in 2:00
Situps	100 in 2:00
Pullups	20
1.5 mile run	under 9:00

    If you need letters of recommendation from SEALs, most SEALs will not endorse you unless you can achieve the above numbers. Do this book two to three times and I guarantee you will be able to hit these scores. Sometimes it takes a solid year of training.

2. **Run in boots and swim with fins!** At least 3-4 months prior to arriving at BUD/S, get the legs used to swimming with fins and running in boots. They issue Bates 924s and UDT or Rocket Fins at BUD/S.

3. **Officers at BUD/S:** Go there ready to lead and get to know your men. Start the team-building necessary to complete BUD/s. You can't do everything by yourself, so learn to delegate but do not be too good to scrub the floors either. Be motivated and push the guys to succeed. Always lead from the front.

4. **Enlisted at BUD/S:** Be motivated and ready to work as a team. Follow orders but provide constant feedback so your team can be better at overcoming obstacles that you will face. Never be late!

5. **BUD/S is six months long!** Prepare for the long term, not the short term. Too many people lose focus early in their training and quit. It would be similar to training for a 10K race and running a Marathon by accident. You have to be mentally focused on running the Marathon—in this case a six month "marathon".

6. **Weekly physical tests:** The four mile timed runs are weekly and occur on the beach—hard packed sand next to the water line. They are tough, but not bad if you prepare properly.

    The 2 mile ocean swims are not bad either if you are used to swimming with fins when you arrive. The obstacle course will get you to if you are not used to climbing ropes and doing pullups. Upper body strength is tested to the max with this test.

7. **Eating at BUD/S:** You get three great meals a day at BUD/S, usually more than you can eat. During Hellweek, you get four meals a day—every six hours! The trick to making it through Hellweek is just make it to the next meal. Break up the week into several six hour blocks of time.

8. **Flutterkicks:** This seems to be a tough exercise for many. Practice 4 count flutterkicks with your ab workouts and shoot for sets of at least 100. There maybe a day you have to do 1000 flutterkicks. By the way—that takes 45 minutes!

9. **Wet and Sandy:** Jumping into the ocean then rolling around in the sand is a standard form of punishment for the class at BUD/S. It is cold and not comfortable, so you just have to prepare yourself for getting wet and sandy everyday at BUD/S. On days that you do not get wet and sandy, it will be the same feeling as getting off early at work on a three day weekend!

10. **Did I mention running?** You should be able to run at least 4 miles in 28 minutes in boots with ease. If not you will so learn to hate the "goon-squad". The goon squad is to motivate you never to be last again or fail a run.

    Any more questions—you can reach me at Stew@stewsmith.com or the www.getfitnow.com website message boards.

HOW TO BECOME
A NAVY SEAL

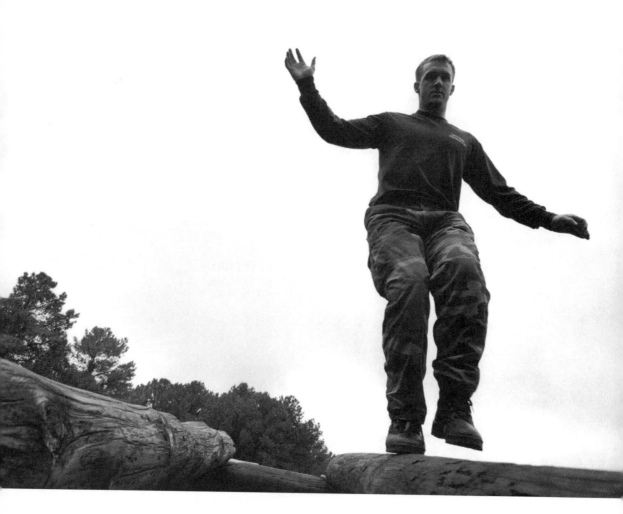

How To Become A Navy SEAL

Becoming a SEAL is challenging. In some cases, it may actually be harder to enter SEAL training than to graduate from SEAL training. This is primarily in the officer ranks, though. Unfortunately, the Navy SEALs do not need officers as much as enlisted personnel, so naturally it will be tougher to become an SEAL officer. The most unusual aspect of SEAL training is that the officers and enlisted participate in the same training. This is very rare in the Navy. In fact it is rare in the entire military. Perhaps this is one reason for the closeness of the SEAL units. It creates an environment of mutual respect.

Before you can enter the SEAL program you must meet the following general requirements:

EYESIGHT: Your eyesight may be no worse than 20/40 in one eye and 20/70 in the other, and it must be correctable to 20/20 with no color blindness. You may have a waiver if vision is 20/70 in one eye and 20/100 in the other, correctable to 20/20. A waiver is also needed for people who get PRK surgery prior to enlisting.

ACADEMIC TESTS: The required ASVAB score is: VE + AR = 104, MC = 50. You may be eligible for a waiver (up to 5 points). Handled on a case-by-case basis.

PHYSICAL TESTS: The BUD/s Physical Fitness Test (PFT)

500 yd sidestroke / breaststroke swim (10:00 rest)

Max pushups in 2:00   (2:00 rest)

Max situps in 2:00   (2:00 rest)

Max pullups   (10:00 rest)

1.5 mile run in boots and pants

AGE: Applications are accepted from men who are 28 years old or less. You may request an age waiver (for those 29-30); however, the age waivers are reviewed on a case-by-case basis.

U.S. CITIZEN: The program is only open to men, and you must be a U.S. citizen for security-clearance requirements.

You can enter into the SEAL program right out of high school at the age of

18 or you can go to college or work and still enlist into the SEAL program up to the age of 28. There are age waivers, but they are few and far between and are handled on a case-by-case basis by the Commanding Officer of BUD/S and the SEAL Community Manager.

Many college graduates enlist instead of entering as an officer mainly due to the large number of officer candidates who apply and the small number who get accepted. The Navy needs more enlisted men than officers in the SEAL Teams basically. Last numbers were one out of every eight who apply get accepted in the officer program.

Another reason why it is challenging to become an officer right out of college is due to the number of college graduates in the enlisted ranks who also place requests for Officer Candidate School. The Navy has a choice of selecting a SEAL veteran enlisted with a college degree or a 22 year old college kid with little experience. That is why many select to enlist right out of college instead of becoming an officer immediately. If you want to be a SEAL, this is a great way to get experience. AND you do not have to go through BUD/s again!

You can enlist either the conventional way or via the SEAL Contract. When you enlist in the U.S. Navy under the SEAL contract, you must sign a contract that states you are giving a certain number of years in return for a guaranteed job. When you enlist under the SEAL Challenge contract, you are guaranteed orders to BUD/S as long as you are qualified and pass a PT screen test in Boot Camp. Everyone who volunteers to take the BUD/S screening test is allowed to take the test at Bootcamp—SEAL Challenge enlisted or the conventional enlisted.

There are advantages to signing the SEAL Challenge Contract. By signing, you are enlisting with the intent of becoming a SEAL. This means that you don't have to worry about getting orders to BUD/S as long as you pass the PT screen test in Boot Camp. This also means that you get four chances to pass the PT screen test at Great Lakes.

If you enlist under any other contract, you are not guaranteed a billet at BUD/S and may have to go to the fleet and complete a minimum tour of duty (which is two years) before requesting an inservice transfer to Naval Special Warfare—BUD/S. You can volunteer at Boot Camp and you may get orders to BUD/S, but it's not guaranteed.

You are also guaranteed an "A" school with the SEAL Challenge, which will give you job-specific training for the rating you choose. We have 22 (technical jobs) to choose from. There are quotas on certain ratings, so they might not all be available when you sign up. Be prepared to be flexible in the job you choose to ensure you can get to BUD/S. If you drop from BUD/S, however, you will work in that rating elsewhere in the Navy. Typically if you quit BUD/S, you can reapply but you will have to spend at least 1-2 years in the Fleet at your rating. **Below is a list of the Navy SEAL ratings to choose from:**

Aviation Boatswain's Mate (AB)

ABs operate, maintain, and repair aircraft catapults, arresting gear, and barricades.

Aviation Ordnanceman (AO)

AOs maintain, repair, install, operate, and handle aviation ordnance equipment.

Aviation Antisubmarine Warfare Operator (AW)

AWs operate airborne radar and electronic equipment used in detecting, locating, and tracking submarines.

Boatswain's Mate (BM)

BMs work in all activities involving deck and boat seamanship, and the maintenance of the ship's external structure and deck equipment.

Electrician's Mate (EM)

EMs operate and repair a ship's or station's electrical power plant and electrical equipment.

Engineman (EN)

Internal combustion engines — diesel or gasoline — maintain refrigeration, air-conditioning, distilling-plant engines, and compressors.

Electronics Technician (ET)

ETs are responsible for electronic equipment used to send and receive messages, detect enemy planes and ships, and determine target distances.

Gunner's Mate (GM)

Navy GMs operate, maintain, and repair all gunnery equipment, guided-missile launching systems, rocket launchers and guns.

Hull Maintenance Technician (HT)

HTs are responsible for maintaining ships' hulls, fittings, piping systems, and machinery to include plumbing and piping systems.

Interior Communications Electrician (IC)

ICs operate and repair electronic devices used in the ship's interior communications systems, SITE TV systems, public address systems, electronic megaphones, and other announcing equipment.

Intelligence Specialist (IS)

An IS is involved in collecting and interpreting intelligence data; analyzing photographs; and preparing charts, maps, and reports that describe in detail the strategic situation all over the world.

Information Systems Technician (IT)

ITs operate the radio/computer communications systems that make complex teamwork possible. They operate radiotelephones and radio-teletypes, administer computer networks and equipment, prepare messages for international and domestic commercial telegraph, and send and receive messages via the Navy system.

Machinist's Mate (MM)

MMs are responsible for the continuous operation of many engines, compressors and gears; refrigeration, air-conditioning, and gas-operated equipment; and other types of machinery afloat and ashore.

Machinery Repairman (MR)

MRs are skilled machine tool operators. They make replacement parts and repair or overhaul a ship's engine auxiliary equipment, such as evaporators, air compressors, and pumps.

Operational Specialist (OS)

OSs operate radar, navigation, and communications equipment in shipboard combat information centers (CICs) or bridges.

Photographer's Mate (PH)

PHs photograph actual and simulated battle operations and make photo records of historic and newsworthy events for the Navy. A five-year enlistment is required.

Personnelman (PN)

PNs provide enlisted personnel with information and counseling about Navy jobs, opportunities for general education and training, promotion requirements, and rights and benefits.

Aircrew Survival Equipmentman (PR)

PRs pack and care for parachutes, as well as service, maintain, and repair flight clothing, rubber life rafts, life jackets, oxygen-breathing apparatus, protective clothing, and air-sea rescue equipment.

Quartermaster (QM)

QMs assist the navigator and officer of the deck (OOD), steer the ship, take radar bearings and ranges, make depth soundings and celestial observations, plot courses, and command small craft.

Storekeeper (SK)

SKs are the Navy's supply clerks. They see that needed supplies are available, including clothing, machine parts, forms, and food. SKs have duties as civilian warehousemen, purchasing agents, stock clerks and supervisors, sales clerks, store managers, buyers, and even fork lift operators.

Signalman (SM)

SMs send and receive various visual messages, handle and route message traffic, operate voice radio, and repair visual signaling devices.

Torpedoman's Mate (TM)

TMs maintain underwater explosive missiles, such as torpedoes and rockets, that are launched from surface ships, submarines and aircraft.

THE PATH TO BUD/S UNDER THE SEAL CHALLENGE CONTRACT:

Once you have successfully taken the ASVAB, selected your RATE, and gotten yourself into peak physical condition, you are ready to sign your SEAL Challenge Contract and enlist in the United States Navy. You can always refer to the Getfitnow.com message boards if you have any questions about what your recruiter is telling you. Sometimes the Navy recruiters do not know what the SEALs do and may not test you physically before you go to Bootcamp. Showing up at Bootcamp out of shape and unable to pass the BUD/s PFT will nullify your orders to BUD/s and you will spend the next 4-5 years in the Fleet—though you can get yourself in shape and lateral transfer after two years.

The most important thing is to keep yourself in top physical shape. You will get four opportunities during boot camp to pass the physical screening test. If you wish to attend BUD/S, you MUST pass the test. The screen test will be given by Navy SEALs at Boot Camp. The SEALs can be found in the Dive Motivator's office at the pool. They will give a Special Warfare brief during your first week at Bootcamp.

After Bootcamp you will attend Navy "A" School, where you learn the basic skills associated with your rate. Continue to work hard and demonstrate leadership qualities. Be sure to continue your physical training. Upon successful completion of "A" School, you are bound for BUD/S. You must be in peak physical condition when you arrive at BUD/s. It is recommend to run in Bates boots (BUD/s Issue) and swim with fins several times a week during "A" school in order to get your legs and ankles prepared for the weekly beach runs and ocean swims.

Before you walk into your local recruiter's office, ensure you have read the previous sections: SEAL Challenge contract, ASVAB, and SEAL source rates. Print out the SEAL Challenge contract which can be downloaded from www.sealchallenge.navy.mil and take it with you to talk to your local recruiter. Once again, there are a few recruiters that may not be 100% knowledgeable of the SEAL Challenge program.

PACKAGE SUBMISSION PROCESS

If you are in the Navy and wish to change jobs and become a SEAL, the requirements for submitting a BUD/S training application package are as follows:

Submit through your chain of command a "Special Request Chit" requesting BUD/S training. Then see your Command Career Counselor to begin the process outlined below.

Submit to SPECWAR/Diver Assignment a "Personnel Action Request" (Form 1306/7). Include the following with your request:

- A certified copy of your ASVAB test scores

- Your physical screening test results

- Pressure and oxygen tolerance test results (if completed)

- Your completed diving physical

- (Form SF88 - SF93)

- Your medical record documenting that all immunizations and HIV results are up to date

- A certified copy of your last performance evaluation report

- Make a copy of your entire package and keep the copy in a safe place.

Mail your package to the address below.

SPECWAR/Diver Assignment
BUPERS PERS401D1
5720 Integrity Drive
Millington, TN 38055-0000
Phone: (901) 874-3622
DSN: 882-3622

You may be an officer or enlisted in another branch of service. There are a few inter-service transfers a year and they are handled on a case by case basis. Many times you have to serve your enlistment with the Marines or Army, get discharged from the service and reapply to the Navy. Most of the time, you do not have to do Bootcamp over again. Your best start on this process is to contact the above number of the SpecWar Detailer in Tennessee.

NEW SPECIAL WARFARE DIVISION IN BOOT CAMP

If you are thinking about joining the SEAL or SWCC communities, the Navy has a great offer for you. Sign up under the SEAL Challenge and specify you want to ship to Great Lakes on a certain date. When you get to boot camp, you will be enrolled in a Special Warfare division with other recruits desiring placement in the Navy's special warfare/special operations communities.

What are the benefits?

You will get the opportunity to PT in preparation for the SEAL/SWCC screen test. (Note: You should be able to pass before going to Bootcamp, which will ensure you don't get out of shape.)

You will wear a special T-shirt denoting your status as a member of the Special Warfare Division.

You will be mentored by members of the Dive Motivator's office to make sure your career is a success.

Special Warfare personnel will give you special briefings on their community.

WHAT DO I HAVE TO DO?

If you are ready to make that all-important decision and enlist, see your local recruiter. If you want to be a SEAL or SWCC, make sure you enlist under the SEAL Challenge. If you aren't ready to enlist by July 2 you can still come into the Navy under the SEAL Challenge contract, which will guarantee that if you can pass the screen test you will go to BUD/S.

How To Become A Navy SEAL

RECRUITERS:

Points of Contact

SEAL Recruiter West Coast
Naval Special Warfare
2446 Trident Way
San Diego, CA 92155-5494
Com. (619) 437-2049 / 437-5009
DSN 577-2049 / 5009
FAX: Com. (619) 437-2018
DSN 577-2018 SEAL Recruiter East Coast

NSWC DET Little Creek
1340 Helicopter Rd.
Norfolk, VA 23521-2945
Com. (757) 363-4128
DSN 864-4128
More information at:
www.getfitnow.com message boards
www.sealchallenge.navy.mil
www.stewsmith.com SEAL Detailer

SPECWAR/Diver Assignment
BUPERS PERS401D1
5720 Integrity Drive
Millington, TN 38055-0000
Com. (901) 874-3622
DSN 882-3622 Dive Motivators (SEAL)
BLDG 1405

Recruit Training Command
Great Lakes, IL 60088
Com. (847) 688-4643
DSN 792-4643
Toll-free Info Line: 1-888-USN-SEAL

For more detailed information about the Navy SEALs contact:
Public Affairs Office
Naval Special Warfare Command
Naval Amphibious Base Coronado
San Diego, CA 92155-5037
(619) 437-3920

MASTERING THE SEAL PHYSICAL FITNESS TEST

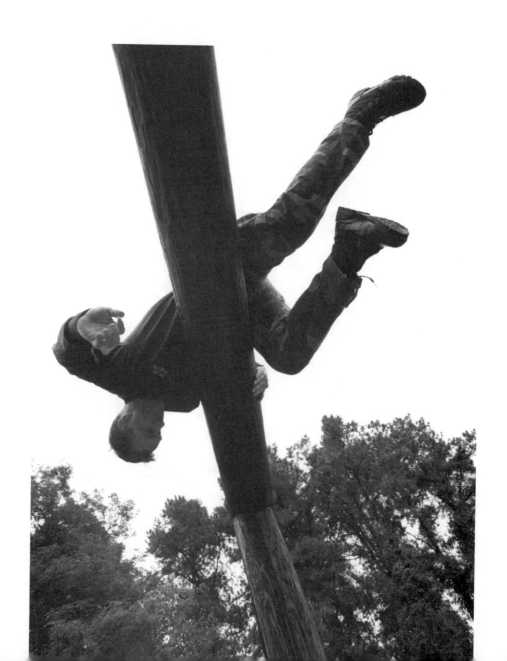

MASTERING THE SEAL PHYSICAL FITNESS TEST!

First of all—the SEAL PFT was developed to test swimming and running capability and upperbody muscle stamina—all of which are vital to becoming a Navy SEAL. The following is designed to help you master the test by demonstrating techniques in training as well as test taking. You need a strategy when taking the SEAL PFT.

Test yourself. The anxiety felt by young SEAL wanna-be's and other service members is largely due to performing within a time limit. The more your workouts are timed the better you are at "pacing" yourself, thus eliminating most anxiety. By practicing the PFT often, you will develop a pace and know when to push yourself at the right times.

THE SWIM:

The 500 yard swim—is what eliminates most people who want to become SEALs. You may pass this part of the test, but you may also completely burn yourself out for the upperbody portion and the run in the process. Here are the test techniques I recommend to score the best time possible while saving your stamina for the pullups, pushups, situps and run:

Kick off the wall and glide as far as you can. You must train using the hypoxic swim pyramid found in this workout to build up your cardiovascular system. You will be winded but you will save yourself several strokes per length.

Strokes per length—the most important factor of the swim. If you can swim a 9:00 swim, that is great. But if it takes you 12-14 strokes per length (25 yards) to do it, you are wasting your energy. On the other hand, if you can swim a 9:00 swim with 6-7 strokes per length you will save over 150 arm strokes and kicks in the process. This is called swimming efficiency! By swimming more efficiently, you will have more energy for the upperbody portion and the run.

How do you get more efficient?

Kick off the wall, double arm pull and glide. Then glide each stroke out after the top arm pull and the kick/recovery to its fullest. Time yourself the old way and then time yourself the new gliding way. You will find that your scores will be the same even though it "feels" like you are swimming slower. You are not swimming slower, you are swimming more efficiently. I recommend an average glide time of 2-3 mississippi's.

PUSHUPS AND PULLUPS—SAME STRATEGY:

Pushups—Placing your hands in the wrong position can seriously affect your maximum score. A perfect location for your hands is just outside shoulder width. This position enables the chest, shoulders and triceps to be equally taxed. Keep hands at shoulder height when in the up position. Your pushups will be weakened if your hands are too low, wide, close or high...in the Navy SEAL pushup test, you are allowed to shake out your arms, as long as one hand and both feet are on the ground. The best way to take this test is to do as many as you can as fast as you can. Then rest in the up position, shake off one arm, repeat with the other arm. Then continue to pump out small sets of 5-10 pushups, shaking it out after every set.

Pullups—During the pullup and pushup test, you want to perform these as fast as possible while adhering to the proper form and technique. The slower you perform these exercises, the more gravity will affect your best score possible. In other words, do not waste your energy returning to the down position. Just let yourself fall. The faster you perform these exercises, the more you will be able to do. Also, look straight up at the sky in order to use your back muscles more for pullups. Pyramid workouts with these exercises will enhance your test scores significantly. The key to training for this part of the test is to keep doing pullups and pushups until you fail. You will succeed in your failure!

SITUPS:

This is an exercise you need to pace. Most people burn out in the first 30 seconds with 30 sit-ups accomplished, only able to perform another 20 or so situps within the next 1:30. By setting a pace at, for instance, 20 situps every 30 seconds, you can turn your score of 50-60 to 80 with very little effort. 25 situps in 30 seconds will give you the score of 100 situps in 2:00.

Mental Games—When I take the test, I always count in my head small numbers like 1-5 or 1-10. I never say eleven or twenty-one. The reason behind this is I feel I am starting over again every time I say "one". This may work for some, it may not. It has helped many in the past.

THE RUN:

For most people the most challenging event of any PFT is by far the run. I receive many requests everyday from military members who are seeking workouts for their 1.5 mile, two or three mile PFT runs (Navy/ Army/Marine Corps respectively). Since all these distances use relatively the same training philosophy—short distance, faster pace—here are a few options to help all Armed Forces members, regardless of service, get a little faster on their runs.

Timed run—PACE—The most important thing is to not start off too fast. Start off too fast and you will burn out and probably fail the run. Learn your pace and set your goal by pacing yourself to the finish. For instance, if your goal is to run the 2 mile run in 14:00, you must run a 7:00 mile or a 1:45 1/4 mile... For you SEAL wanna-be's, if you want to run a 9:00 1.5 mile test score, you need to start out and finish with a 90 second 1/4 mile. Keep this pace and you will have a 9:00 score.

Recommended workout and techniques—The Four Mile Track Workout has worked for many military and short distance runners for years. This workout is basically interval training. Interval training means you run at a certain pace for a particular distance then increase the pace for the same distance.

The Four Mile Track Workout is broken into 1/4 mile sprints and jogs and 1/8 mile sprints and jogs for a total of four miles. The workout goes as follows:

4 Mile Track Work

    Jog—1 mile in 7:00 - 8:00

Three sets of:

    Sprint-1/4 mile

    Jog—1/4 mile in 1:45

Six sets of:

    Sprint-1/8 mile

    Jog—1/8 mile 1:00

Do this workout without walking to rest. The only rest you will receive is during your slower jogging pace. Try to catch your breath while you jog. Have fun with this one; it is tough.

Another good speed workout is called REPEATS. Simply run a certain distance as fast as you can a specified number of times. This time you get to walk to recover and catch your breath before the next sprint. You can try one of the following distances for a challenging workout:

Mile repeats

1 mile x 3-4 (walk 1/2 mile in between) = 3-4 miles

1/2 mile repeats—

1/2 mile x 6 (walk 1/4 mile in between) = 3 miles

1/4 mile repeats—

1/4 mile repeats x 12 (walk 1/8 mile in between) = 3 miles

1/8 mile repeats—

1/8 mile repeat x 16 (walk 100 yds in between) = 2 miles

Finally, if you have not had enough, you can try mixing shorter jogs and sprints together for a longer period of time. This type of training is great for building the speed and endurance needed for any of the PFTs or 5 or 10K races. I call them SPRINT / JOGS. Simply run about 50 yards as fast as you can then jog 50 yards fairly slow in order to catch your breath. I like doing this one where telephone poles line the road so I can just sprint to one telephone pole then jog to the next.

Sprint / Jogs

50 yd sprint / 50 yd jog for 10, 20, 30 minutes

All of these workouts are fantastic ways to get faster but build the needed endurance which most sprinters lack. Remember to take big deep breaths, relax your upperbody and slightly bend your arms. Do not run flat footed.

These are the techniques to ace the SEAL PFT and any other physical fitness test. Many members of the FBI, Marine RECON, Army Special Forces and Navy SEALs have utilized these techniques and went from wanna-be to their dream job. Good luck. If you have any questions, you can reach me on the www.getfitnow.com web boards or at stew@stewsmith.com

ABOUT THE AUTHOR

Lt. Stewart G. "Stew" Smith graduated from the United States Naval Academy in 1991. After graduation, he received orders to Basic Underwater Demolition/SEAL (BUD/S) training (Class 182). While on the SEAL teams, he learned to achieve maximum levels of physical fitness thanks to the knowledge of several Chief Petty Officer SEALs, Navy doctors, and nutritionists.

Over half of Stew Smith's life has been devoted to athletics and exercise. From grade school to SEAL training, he has learned and developed several different training regimens. **The Complete Guide to Navy SEAL Fitness** is a reflection of Stew's knowledge and drive to succeed.

After four years on the SEAL Teams, Stew was stationed at the Naval Academy and put in charge of the physical training and selection of future BUD/S students. Since 1995, LT. Stew Smith's use of this workout program has yielded amazing results. The workouts he developed to prepare students for SEAL training are still in use today by SEAL recruiters (The BUD/S Warning Order). And, of the more than thirty students that Stew has sent to BUD/S, not a single man has quit and all have stated that they were physically prepared.

TAKE YOUR FITNESS TO THE MAX!

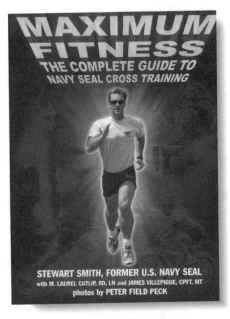

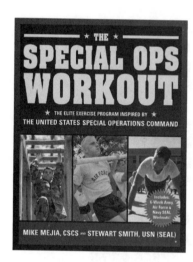

OFFICIAL MILITARY WORKOUT GUIDES!

Add these authorized books to your collection!
Learn the secrets to what keeps America's Armed Forces
in fighting shape!

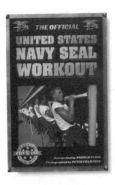 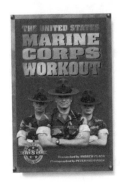

THE OFFICIAL U.S.
NAVY SEAL WORKOUT
ISBN 1-57826-009-4
$14.95

THE OFFICIAL U.S.
MARINE CORPS WORKOUT
ISBN 1-57826-011-6
$14.95

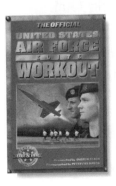 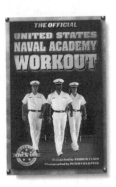

THE OFFICIAL U.S.
AIR FORCE ELITE WORKOUT
ISBN 1-57826-029-9
$14.95

THE OFFICIAL U.S.
NAVAL ACADEMY WORKOUT
ISBN 1-57826-010-8
$14.95

Available wherever books are sold, or direct from the publisher.

Toll-free orders 1-800-906-1234
Order online at www.getfitnow.com

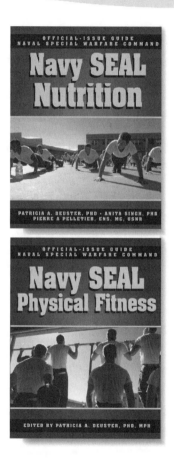